Being Fertile

10 Steps to help you overcome the
struggles of infertility, get
pregnant, and create a happy,
healthy family

Dr. Spence Pentland

Disclaimer

The information contained in this book is intended to provide accurate and helpful health information for the general public. It is made available with the understanding that the author and publisher are not engaged in rendering specific individualized medical, health, psychological, or any other kind of personal professional services, diagnosis, or treatment recommendations. The information should not be considered complete and does not cover all diseases, ailments, physical conditions or their treatment. It should not be used in place of a call or visit to a medical, health or other competent professional, who should be consulted before adopting any of the suggestions in this book or drawing inferences from it. Dr. Spence Pentland specifically disclaims all responsibility for any liability, loss or risk, personal or otherwise, which is incurred as a consequence, directly or indirectly, of the use and application of any of the material in this book.

www.yinstill.com

ISBN: 978-1508900337

Book cover design by Carolyn Sheltraw
Illustrations by Ian Drew Pentland

This book is dedicated to my family.

Words cannot describe how much I love you all.

~Spence

How to Use This Book

1. Do not simply read through the pages of this book - study it, consume it, absorb it. Write in the columns and blank pages, highlight, underline, star, dog ear, and flag pages that are important to you. Treat this book like it is something you are going to have to teach to others when you are done.

2. Be sure to complete the exercises at the end of each step. These will serve you as a guide for moving forward on your journey toward family. Ink it, don't just think it. Then re-write in a separate journal and share your plan with someone who can help hold you accountable.

3. Review weekly. Document actions taken and rate your progress and accomplishments. Do this for at least 3 months, 6 to 12 being ideal. Revisit the pages of the book when you feel necessary and revise your plan where needed.

4. Finally, pay it forward. When your time with this book is complete, gift it to someone else in need or donate it to your local women's centre or library.

I wish you all the best with creating your family.

~Spence

Foreword

As Reproductive Endocrinologists, many aspects of the care we provide patients in achieving pregnancy are not based in strong scientific evidence. We are faced with a variety of clinical situations that simply merit common sense and a conservative approach. Modern fertility treatments like in vitro fertilization (IVF) are increasingly more effective, but as artificial methods of conception, they expose mother and child to a number of risks during and after pregnancy. Proudly we now have the ability to provide the vast majority of our patients with a successful pregnancy, but not without exposing them to hazards inherent in the treatments. Given this, we must be clear on the diagnosis and supportive of any Complementary or Alternative Medicine (CAM) treatment that can provide for a natural conception or improvement in the effectiveness of our treatment.

The scientific evidence for the use of many CAM treatments are mixed at best, with most focus placed on the use of acupuncture. Many aspects of these treatments and interventions do not lend themselves to scientific methods of study, so will likely never be validated. However, I believe that certain CAM therapies, such as acupuncture, can be helpful in the management of infertility.

The level of stress that our patients undergo during their struggles with infertility is commonly overlooked. It is estimated that 12% of infertile women are clinically depressed (Peterson, 2014), and up to 23% have generalized anxiety disorder (Chen, 2004). Using psychological measures of mental health, infertility has been shown to generate similar levels of stress as major cancer (Domar, 1993). Not unexpectedly, this stress also results in more long-term marital discourse and divorce (Gameriro, 2011). In terms of IVF and other advanced treatments, we do our best to reduce anxiety levels by making ourselves available to patients and streamlining the process to minimize any disruption to daily lives, however, the treatment can be very stressful for some. Treatment outcomes with IVF may be lower when stress levels are high (Quant, 2013), so any intervention that helps relax our patients (i.e., acupuncture) will certainly be of benefit. At the very least, the delicate medical procedures required for IVF will be easier to perform on a patient that is less stressed or "in her zone".

Many of our patients find value in yoga, meditation and exercise during fertility treatment and throughout pregnancy. Traditional Chinese Medicine (TCM) practitioners help our patients by providing not just acupuncture, but also a variety of life-style modifications that assist with weight loss and stress relief. Optimizing one's health is important for success with both natural conception and fertility treatments. To optimize outcomes with fertility treatments and pregnancy outcome, the physicians at Pacific Centre for Reproductive Medicine (PCRM) advocate a healthy lifestyle. This includes the use of dietary supplements, a healthy balanced diet, maintenance of a normal body weight and physical activity.

Dr. Pentland is a pioneer in the field of reproductive care and one of a few that delivers his care with knowledge of both TCM and assisted reproductive technologies. He also faces the challenges of infertility with a scientific mind and has always supported research and academics at PCRM. He works tirelessly for his patients and makes himself available for all aspects of care, whether medical or emotional. Yinstill has been a pleasure to work with and their approach on all levels has been highly ethical and unobtrusive. Over the years, our practices have slowly integrated and are now at a point where patients can seamlessly experience the benefits of both therapies. In 2011, Dr. Pentland established the IVF Acupuncture group at PCRM to make CAM more accessible to our patients, and are currently publishing our successes with this unique collaborative model for the management of infertility. For the integration of general fertility care, little correspondence between us is required as we have become more comfortable with each other's approach. I have had the pleasure of working closely with Dr. Pentland for almost a decade. Together we have helped hundreds women and couples to experience the magic of children. As parents ourselves, we can think of no feeling comparable in this world, and given what we do for a living, a gift that we will never take for granted.

Jeff Roberts, MD FRCS
Co-Director, Pacific Centre for Reproductive Medicine
Assistant Clinical Professor, Departments of OBGYN and Pharmacology and Therapeutics & Anesthesia, University of British Columbia

Table of Contents

Prologue

I have learned so much over the past 10 years treating women and couples that are trying to start or expand on their families and I am eager and excited to share these experiences in this book.

Within the clinical setting, every consultation with each woman or couple is a breeding ground for deeply individualized recommendations to improve health and fertility. It is an intimate process of connection and trust, woven together with the nuances of Traditional Chinese Medicine (TCM).

I hope the pages that follow capture some of that connection, speak to you, inspire hope and give you a clear glimpse into the tools that can be used to change the trajectory of your life, and possibly help you in creating your own happy healthy family.

Not unlike the fundamentals of TCM, I believe that the cultivation of fertility is not a complicated journey, yet understandably, can seem profound when searching for *your own personal* solution. There are no magic bullets, no shortcuts and very few quick fixes.

I decided to keep this book as straightforward as possible with 10 chapters representing the 10 steps that I explore at great depth with each woman or couple that come to my clinic. Taking the time to really care for yourself, accepting your circumstances and having faith that you will reach your goal through perseverance is the basis for success when faced with the difficulties of starting a family.

What really makes myself and the other doctors at our

clinic, Yinstill Reproductive Wellness, stand apart is our integration and collaboration with Vancouver's largest IVF centres. These relationships over the years have deepened my understanding of what the women I see are going through, and how to better support them on their journey.

I am very proud to be part of the team of professionals at Yinstill. We are all dedicated to raising the bar in the field of complementary and alternative reproductive medicine. I encourage you to take some time to read the many testimonials on our website (yinstill.com) from the women and couples we have worked with over the years, as their stories in their words may help you understand the work that is being done and how it could help you.

I want to thank you for deciding to read this book. It demonstrates the dedication you have toward creating your family. The struggles you may be going through can be extremely difficult and your perseverance and strength is honorable. I urge you to keep doing everything in your power to stay the course and maintain faith that your dreams will come true.

Biography

A bit about me...

My name is Spence Pentland and my mission is to optimize the health of my clients and increase their chances of conception in order to build happy families because to me, nothing is more important than family.

I am a licenced Doctor of Traditional Chinese Medicine (http://ctcma.bc.ca), a Fellow of the American Board of Oriental Reproductive Medicine (http://aborm.org), and a member of the Canadian Association of Oriental Obstetrical Medicine (http://caoom.org).

Since 2004, my clinical practice in Vancouver, British Columbia has focused exclusively on the treatment of men's and women's reproductive health, specifically fertility and its related conditions including polycystic ovary syndrome (PCOS), endometriosis, and recurrent pregnancy loss (RPL). We support women and couples going through In Vitro Fertilization (IVF) with the goals of increasing pregnancy rates and reducing stress along the journey. Lastly, we care for women throughout their pregnancies, helping prevent miscarriage, alleviating common complaints, and preparing them for labour and delivery.

After pursuing undergraduate studies in botany, herbal medicine, horticulture, psychology and philosophy, I went on to graduate with my doctor of TCM (Dr. TCM) from the acclaimed International College of Traditional Chinese Medicine in Vancouver before completing my internship at Anhui Hospital of TCM in Hefei City, China. In 2008, I obtained certification with the American Board of Oriental

Reproductive Medicine (ABORM).

I am the founder of The IVF Acupuncture Group of Greater Vancouver, operating 7 days a week for on-site embryo transfer day acupuncture treatments. I am also a member of IAAC (Infertility Awareness Association), CFAS (Canadian Fertility and Andrology Society), and ASRM (American Society for Reproductive Medicine).

In collaboration with Dr. Jeff Roberts of the Pacific Centre for Reproductive Medicine (PCRM), I am completing clinical research on the stress-reducing effects of acupuncture when used in conjunction with IVF. This is currently in the process of being accepted for presentation at the Pacific Coast Reproductive Society (PCRS) annual general meeting in California.

The environment and its impact on our health is a passion of mine. My family and our company donate regularly to The David Suzuki Foundation, The Canadian Association of Physicians for the Environment (CAPE), Vancouver Farmer's Markets, and Health Action Network Society (HANS). We also plant a tree for every baby our clinic plays a role in bringing into this world, every baby who doesn't make it into the world, and for everyone that helps Yinstill grow. We call this 'The Yinstill Gratitude Forest'. Locally, we give to an organization that supports pregnant women and new mothers who need a helping hand. Internationally, we are proud to support Shanti Uganda, a birthing centre in Africa that helps prevent hundreds of mother and baby birth-related deaths each year.

As the former president of the Traditional Chinese Medicine Association of British Columbia and the provincial TCM quality assurance committee, I remain active in educating healthcare colleagues and the public on the powerful benefits of Traditional Chinese Medicine (TCM) and acupuncture, working steadily on the

4

integration of ancient Daoist wisdom into modern western life as a way to build awareness about reproductive health.

When not helping others start their families, I can be found spending time with my beautiful wife, Chantal, and my two amazing sons. After getting married and having my two boys, Salix and Ari, I was gifted with an intimate understanding of what each and every client that comes through the clinic door is in search of and I desperately want each and every woman and couple to have the chance to be graced with the heart-opening love that children bring.

I absolutely love working with people trying to start or expand their family. When someone I've been working with tells me a baby is on the way, the feeling I get is hard to put into words, but it confirms for me that I'm doing exactly what I'm supposed to be doing.

Introduction

If you were baking a cake for someone you loved on a special occasion, you would take great care to follow the recipe, right? You would preheat the oven and use the best quality ingredients, you would stir and whip and measure with the utmost of care before baking it at just the right temperature and watching it mindfully. And the results would be magnificent and worth the effort.

But that's just a cake...

The subject of this book is how to create the most precious thing of all--a human life, so I trust you will want to heed an even greater regard for the recipe at hand. I have included 10 steps, each one as important as the next. I cannot guarantee with absolute certainty that you will reach your goal. My experience has shown me time and again that these steps will greatly improve your chances. If you follow them, you will improve your physical and emotional health and provide the best possible environment for your unborn child.

It is a great privilege for me to share my knowledge with you as we embark on the most important and rewarding journey of your life. I wish you happy and healthy children and to know the joys of being a parent in whatever way that comes to you.

Let's get started, shall we?

Step One

Ancient Healing:

An Overview of Traditional Chinese Medicine

A mediocre doctor treats disease, a good doctor prevents disease and a master doctor teaches his community to be well.
~Huang Di Nei Jing Su Wen

ince this is a book based in Traditional Chinese Medicine (TCM) and I am a doctor of TCM, I think an overview of its basic philosophy and ideas is a good place to start.

With explanations of the fundamental principles including patterns and their symptoms, treatment of these patterns through acupuncture and herbs and accompanying case studies, I aim to give you an understanding of what it is that I do and how it can help you achieve your dream of having a baby.

One of the key components of TCM that differentiates it from western medicine is that the body, mind and spirit are not separate from each other. Your emotions, sleep patterns, stress levels, relationships, job satisfaction and personal fulfillment for example, are all connected to your health and your ability to conceive a child. TCM looks at you as a whole individual, diagnosing your patterns of disharmony and treating you accordingly. You will never leave the office of a doctor of TCM with a diagnosis of 'unexplained infertility'. There is an explanation for your reproductive challenges and I am fully invested in helping you discover what that is and overcoming it.

There is never a wrong time to begin to utilize the powers of TCM to aid in your fertility journey. When women and couples come to see me, they are at one of three places; **1.** they want to optimize their chances of natural conception before any type of western medical intervention, **2.** they want support while going through western medical assisted reproductive technologies, or **3.** they have exhausted all western medical options and have turned to TCM as their last hope.

TCM is very much a partnership. Rather than *telling* you what is happening within *your* body, I will guide you through self-monitoring so that we can co-develop a plan that is tailored to you and addresses all areas of wellness - not only the symptom of infertility. The human body is highly intelligent and will tell you everything you need to know if you listen carefully.

The four ancient pillars of TCM pattern diagnosis are looking, listening/smelling, questioning and palpation (touch). By utilizing these simple and trusted techniques, an accurate foundation for diagnosis is identified so that specific acupuncture points, custom herbal formulations and individual lifestyle recommendations can be made.

Maintaining and restoring balance are at the heart of diagnosis and treatment in TCM and there are two primary tools used to do this: acupuncture and herbal medicine. While they are intricate and take years to master, the basic ideology is that acupuncture opens and herbal medicine heals.

What IS Acupuncture and Herbal Medicine?

Acupuncture

Acupuncture is based on the premise that we have energy meridians running through our bodies which gives power to our nervous system and provides our organic physical being with fundamental life force. When this energy or 'Qi' (pronounced 'chee') is blocked or not flowing smoothly, it causes a variety of problems including infertility. Using a series of very tiny needles at key points throughout your body restores the flow of energy and aids the body in returning to its natural state of perfect health.

Acupuncture is not a drug, nor does it override physiology; instead, it promotes the body's regular circulation and rhythms so that it can function unimpeded. Your body's innate desire is to be balanced and healthy. Acupuncture gives it a helping hand. Like stitches for a deep cut, acupuncture addresses deep programming and allows the body to do what it was designed to do: be well. While it's not the actual healer, it creates an optimal environment for the body to do its own healing, not unlike stitches.

Benefits of Acupuncture

- *Optimizes natural fertility potential by correcting conditions that may be contributing to difficulties with conception. It is also utilized by those who are proactive and simply want to be at their pinnacle of health before conceiving and carrying a pregnancy.*
- *Improves pregnancy and live birth rates, as well as reducing miscarriage and ectopic pregnancy rates when used in conjunction with In Vitro Fertilization (IVF). There is a burgeoning body of research to support this. Refer to Step Nine for a more extensive discussion and references*

11

regarding TCM and how it helps improves IVF success.

- *Improves blood circulation to the reproductive organs and thickens the uterine lining (for more things that you can do at home to enhance blood flow to the reproductive organs, see Step Eight). Blood delivers nutrition and oxygen to every cell, as well as carrying away waste. In the case of IVF, the possibility of enhanced delivery of IVF medications to the developing eggs via optimized blood flow is a well-accepted theory.*

- *Reduces stress and anxiety. Besides the effect acupuncture has on improving blood flow to the reproductive organs, this is likely the most accepted reason the Reproductive Endocrinologists (fertility & IVF doctors) send their patients to me. Its effect on reducing the tone or excitability of the sympathetic nervous system is well documented, reported by patients and observed time and time again in the clinical setting. This change in the nervous system further increases blood flow to the reproductive organs.*

- *Helps restore hormonal balance involved in all aspects of reproductive and whole body functioning (i.e. thyroid, insulin, estrogen, FSH-follicle stimulating hormone, progesterone, testosterone, adrenal).*

- *Regulates the menstrual cycle and induces regular ovulation by balancing hormones, helping with weight loss and removing emotional blockages (such as in women struggling with PCOS).*

- *Regulates immune function required for implantation and preventing miscarriage. The body's delicate wisdom needs to be given the space to function as needed here. Too much or too little immune response may result in repeated implantation failure. If you suffer from allergies or atopic conditions like asthma, eczema, sinusitis or recurrent early pregnancy loss, then immune regulation should be an important health goal.*

- *Supports women suffering from recurrent pregnancy loss (RPL) on an emotional level. TCM can help reduce the fear of trying to conceive or being pregnant and boost the willpower necessary to once again move forward. It may also help mend the broken heart that accompanies these losses.*
- *Reduces pain and inflammation in conditions such as Vulvodynia (pelvic pain) and Endometriosis.*
- *Can improve sperm quality such as motility, count, morphology, and possibly DNA fragmentation rates (see Step Ten for more information on the treatment of male factor infertility).*
- *Enhances sexual function and desire, which so often becomes major obstacles after trying to conceive for a period of time.*
- *Eases the discomforts of pregnancy. Reduction of nausea, aches and pains, hypertension, headaches and many other symptoms observed in the clinic. The management of gestational diabetes, turning breech babies, and preparing the woman and the cervix for labour are also common applications.*

Chinese Herbal Medicine

Using plants to heal the body is nothing new. While to some they are considered an alternative, in fact, plants are the original ingredients of westernized medicine as we know it today. Without the extraction and isolation of one single component of the plant, or the addition of synthetics and fillers, herbs are just medicine in its unadulterated state. They can be used in conjunction with acupuncture or on their own. Sometimes they will be in capsules or tablets, but often they will be prescribed in teas to maximize potency. They may be foul-tasting to the unaccustomed palate but tantalizing the taste buds is not the goal. There may be a little pain but there is much to gain!

Benefits of Chinese Herbal Medicine

- *Aids a dietary cleanse, digestion, appetite control, and weight management.*
- *Gently encourages the body's systems to move toward balance and optimal functioning.*
- *Increases blood circulation and helps remove blockages such as blood clots and cysts.*
- *Soothes emotions, sedates mental activity and reduces stress. Particularly effective in the premenstrual phase.*
- *Balances body fluid metabolism, helping reduce the retention of water and enhance elimination of waste.*
- *Boosts resistance to viral and bacterial attacks and helps reduce inflammation via immune system regulation.*
- *Warms the body if too cold; cools the body if too warm.*
- *Regulates the bowels and urinary function, optimizing the elimination of waste.*
- *Improves sleep conditions such as trouble falling asleep, light sleep, night sweats and waking early with difficulty going back to sleep.*
- *Helps in the management of painful conditions such as Endometriosis.*
- *Supplements deficiencies of vital energy and nourishes blood production.*
- *Helps stop unwanted bleeding as is the case with fibroids, polyps or the flooding that may occur as a result of hormonal shifting toward the end of a woman's reproductive years.*
- *Regulates the menstrual cycle including ovulation and PMS via the restoration of hormonal balance.*
- *Is traditionally used to 'secure fetus' and reduce the incidence of miscarriage.*
- *Improves sperm parameters most notably by reducing the TCM pattern of Heat* (sperm's #1*

enemy) that so many men present with.
- *Increases libido (both male and female) and helps manage erectile dysfunction and premature ejaculation.*

* While there may be parallels between TCM terminology and western medical conditions (i.e., Heat=inflammation), direct correlations aren't always the case and it's best to seek a professional opinion.

Wondering what it will cost?

The average cost of a private acupuncture treatment in North America ranges from $70-$100, and Chinese herbal medicine can vary drastically depending on quality, method of administration and dose, but in general will be between $100-$300 per month.

You could estimate weekly acupuncture treatments for one year (52) at $85 = $4420 and daily Chinese herbal medicine for twelve months at $200 per month = $2400. So for a full year of consistent acupuncture and Chinese herbal medicine, you would pay approximately $6,820.

This sum is considerably less than an average IVF cycle. In addition to the profound effects on your health and well-being, you are greatly increasing your chances of conception and a healthy child with TCM.

Most extended medical plans in Canada cover acupuncture treatment.

If you have the gift of time and you're not rushing to conceive, preparing your body before pregnancy with TCM is a wise move...a decision I dream that every potential parent would make. It is becoming well accepted that the health of the mother and the father before conception plays a role in determining the health their child will experience throughout life. Being healthy preconception may be the best gift you can give your child.

TCM Pattern Identification

It is my belief that the western world could benefit significantly by learning the basic theories of TCM because while structured and scientific, it is a beautiful and artistic way of interpreting the human body and achieving health.

TCM pattern identification is a system of diagnosis that organizes the signs and symptoms a person is presenting so that appropriate diet and lifestyle coaching, acupuncture points and Chinese herbal medicine can be administered.

Some of the terminology you'll hear referenced in TCM may be unfamiliar. Below is a simplified version of the types of diagnosis and what they mean as well as case studies for better understanding.

NOTE: *People often exhibit two or more of these patterns simultaneously and that seemingly conflicting patterns may appear in different parts of the body. For example, hot and cold or damp and dry. This is normal and why a licenced Doctor of TCM should properly diagnose you before any conclusions are drawn through self-diagnosis.*

Heat

General Features: Red skin eruptions like rashes, eczema and acne, constipation with dry stool, anxiety, red tongue with yellow coating, rapid pulse rate, restlessness, easy agitation and anger, high blood pressure, red face, bleeding from the nose or anus, bad breath, canker sores, feeling hot, disliking heat, fever, inflammation, dark yellow urine and a thirst for cold drinks.

Gynecological Features: Heat can manifest as short cycles

(less than 26 days) with thicker blood consistency that is bright or dark red in colour and heavy volume. Bleeding may occur outside regular times as in premenstrual spotting. There may also be a lack of cervical fluid.

Interpretations: Heat may appear as inflammation or an overactive immune response, as is the case with allergies. A person with excess heat might experience high stress and anxiety and be an overachiever. Dehydration can become an issue, particularly if excessive amounts of coffee are relied on for energy. Excesses of male hormones may be present such as with PCOS or hyperthyroidism.

Heat Example
Melanie

- **general info** - Melanie was a 31-year-old lawyer trying to conceive for one year. Her husband was 43 and traveled a lot. Since coming off her IUD one year prior, her cycles had been irregular in length.
- **history** - She admitted to being controlling and smiled with the knowledge that surrendering was an important part of her journey toward family. She emphasized that she was not the type of person to relax so I emphasized that relaxing would be one of our primary goals for treatment. She was extremely active, which may have contributed to her irregular cycles as well as allergies and childhood illnesses that may also have played a role. She reported that her husband's being away a lot, financial debt and work were all major stressors in her life. All medical testing for both she and her husband came back without issue.
- **presentations** - She had irregular cycles ranging from 26-42 days with a very light menstrual flow and severe pain during periods with many premenstrual symptoms. She was very thin, typically held herself in closed postures and rarely

smiled. Heartburn, eczema, aversion to heat and palpitations were present and she had multiple allergies and digestive problems.

- **pattern(s)** - According to TCM, Heat affecting the Heart was prominent. This was caused by Liver Qi Stagnation. There was also a pattern of Kidney Yang deficiency/cold resulting in Heart Kidney disharmony. Blood Stasis and Blood deficiency patterns were also displaying but of secondary importance.
- **goals** - Our primary goal was to address the length of her menstrual cycle length and its blood volume. We also worked on improving urinary frequency, stress, heartburn, palpitations, her aversion to heat, allergies, the condition of her skin, sweet cravings, gas, bloating, abdominal pain, painful periods, cervical mucous and PMS. Her ability to surrender and accept what was happening was vital to the outcome.
- **recommendations & treatment** -
  - Acupuncture once a week and a mild dose of Chinese herbal tablets
  - Decreasing coffee consumption and foods that may have been causing inflammation
  - Reducing exercise slightly
  - Paying attention to body signs that indicated ovulation rather than relying on temperature or ovulation strips
  - Having conversations with her husband about the stressors in her life and asking for help
  - Taking CoQ10 and fish oils daily
  - Accepting and surrendering to her circumstances
  - Chiropractic treatments to address her misaligned pelvic structure
- **outcome** - The first couple of months that we worked together, she had 30-day cycles with an increase in menstrual volume. She soon reported a major improvement in her digestive function

which at the beginning inhibited her from taking all the recommended supplements and Chinese herbal medicine, but that improved very quickly. She tried a couple of rounds of Clomid (or clomiphene citrate, an oral medication used to help a woman ovulate) which were unsuccessful. After a TCM treatment course of 14 weeks, she decided to take a break from trying to conceive. Two months later, she contacted me to inform me that she was happily 8 weeks pregnant. Her pregnancy was without complication and she delivered a healthy baby boy.

- **cost** - Approximately $1,500 (included; 3.5 months of weekly acupuncture treatments, daily Chinese herbal tablets and recommended dietary supplements).

Dampness

Features: Slightly overweight, sluggish in overall energy and movement, water retention, loose bowel movements, gas and bloating, fatigue after eating, candida or yeast infections, achy joints, wet tongue, soggy pulse, painful ovulation, stringy mucous in menstrual blood.

Gynecological Features: An accumulation of dampness can manifest as blockage which causes long cycles (35 days) and watery discoloured blood. Painful ovulation and stringy mucous in menstrual blood are also signs of dampness.

Interpretations: In general, the Damp person has dietary and/or digestive issues and quite likely favors starchy carbohydrates and sugary sweets often due to emotional eating. Fatigue inhibits regular exercise. The lack of exercise and emotional eating often result in weight issues and water retention causing a puffy appearance. They may be difficult to motivate and lazy, the opposite of Yin deficient.

19

Dampness (Phlegm) Example
Adrienne

- **general info** - Adrienne was a 33 year-old overweight woman with irregular cycles. She often did not ovulate on her own and showed many other characteristics congruent with PCOS. She had been trying to conceive for 14 months when she decided to try TCM.

- **history** - Very irregular ovulation and menses most often brought on by progesterone. Some of her cycles were over 100 days and her basal body temperature was also erratic. Most of her medical testing (thyroid, androgens, glucose) was within range but borderline.

- **presentations** - Irregular cycles, overweight, allergies (asthma, sinusitis, foggy mind), digestive issues (bloating, abdominal pain, heartburn), poor sleep, sweats easily, headaches, restlessness, cankers and acne.

- **pattern(s)** - According to TCM, Adrienne is most prominently displaying a Damp/Phlegm pattern. This is causing blockage of necessary functions which regulate ovulation. This pattern is the result of an underlying Qi deficiency and Qi stagnation. Also, due to this blockage, mild Heat is resulting.

- **goals** - Optimizing her reproductive health and fertility by inducing regular ovulation and regulating menstrual cycles. Weight loss through changing dietary habits and improvement of digestion. Regulating allergies and associated symptoms and increasing her sleep quality.

- **recommendations & treatment** -
    - Weekly acupuncture treatments and daily Chinese herbal medicine
    - Dietary cleanse for one month
    - Eliminating gluten and dairy and drinking more water
    - An overall focus on a whole food plant-based

diet
- Hot foot soaks before bed
- Increased fat burning activity
- Implementing an earlier bed time
- Taking fish oils, Vitamin D and inositol daily supplements

- **outcome** - After 3 months of consistent treatment with acupuncture and with the aid of Clomid, she became pregnant. Unfortunately, this ended in an early miscarriage. We continued with regular acupuncture and incorporated Chinese herbal medicine as well as dietary supplements. She displayed a drastic improvement in allergies and her cycles started to regulate. Her commitment to good diet and exercise never failed. After 37 acupuncture treatments within 10 months and approximately six months of Chinese herbal medicine without the use of Clomid, she ended up falling pregnant again and carrying to term, giving birth to a healthy baby boy.

- **cost** - Approximately $4,500 (included 10 months of weekly acupuncture, daily Chinese herbal medicine for five months and recommended dietary supplements).

Yin Deficiency

Features: Night sweats, hot flashes, thin body, lack of bodily fluids, restlessness, flushed cheeks, light sleep and a persistent gnawing hunger.

Gynecological Features: Light volume of menstrual blood and cervical mucous that can lead to absence of ovulation and menstruation.

Interpretations: The phrase 'burning the candle at both ends' applies to this person. They are often restless with a lot on their minds, hence the difficulty shutting down properly at night to rest. These people tend to be quite rigid in character and may look tired or withered.

Yin Deficiency Example
Summer
- **general info** - Summer was a 38 year-old health care professional diagnosed with high FSH and diminished ovarian reserve (DOR). Originally she came to see me to optimize her chances of success with her upcoming IVF cycle. Her first child was conceived via IVF.
- **history** - FSH high, antral follicle count low and a diminished ovarian reserve. She'd had her first child via IVF two years ago. She had previously been slightly overactive with exercise but had cut back. While consistently undergoing acupuncture treatments, she went through two back-to-back IVF cycles within five months, the first resulting in an early miscarriage at five weeks. The first stimulated four follicles and the second only two, with one fertilized and transferred on day three post egg retrieval. She decided to take a break and regroup before doing another possible IVF cycle. This was when we implemented Chinese herbal medicine to restore balance and improve reproductive potential.
- **presentations** - Thin athletic-type body, night sweats and poor sleeping habits in general, scanty clotted menses, extreme emotional stress in the form of anxiety, fear and irritability, especially with her husband. Bowels that alternated between loose to constipated, multiple premenstrual symptoms, multiple digestive complaints, eczema and low libido.
- **pattern(s)** - According to TCM, Summer primarily displayed Yin deficiency. She also had a clear pattern of Qi Stagnation. Both Yin deficiency and Qi stagnation were creating Heat, which may have been responsible for the high FSH and difficulties stimulating with IVF medications.

- **goals** - To optimize her reproductive health and fertility by alleviating night sweats, soothing the emotional stress in her life, regulating bowel movements and digestion, increasing menstrual volume and reducing clotted menses.
- **recommendations & treatment** – Unwavering commitment to weekly acupuncture appointments and daily Chinese herbal medicine. My plan was to systematically reduce the number of tasks she was doing daily in regards to her 'fertility' enhancement.
- **outcome** - After 33 acupuncture treatments (supporting two full IVF cycles) and only three months of taking Chinese herbal medicine (and deciding against more IVF), Summer became much more relaxed, displayed a drastic increase in cervical mucous and sleep quality, an increase in PMS (which can sometimes be a positive biomarker for improved hormonal function in women of advanced maternal age) and fell pregnant, naturally! She went on to have a beautiful baby boy.
- **cost** - Approximately $3,300 (included eight months of weekly acupuncture treatments, recommended dietary supplements and Chinese herbal medicine for three months).

Commentary - *This is a classic case of a woman who was doing too much, trying to accomplish pregnancy versus taking the steps necessary to receive pregnancy. She was a 'doer' and because of this was a very accomplished woman, respected by all those around her as being 'the one that knows'. It was only when she decided to step back from trying so hard, stop convincing herself that IVF is the only way she could become pregnant, let her body's innate wisdom shine through and take a course of reproductive-enhancing Chinese herbal medicine, that she was finally in a place to allow pregnancy to occur and it did. We became very close with* *each session consisting of profound conversations about her deeper inner needs and requirements for holistic health.*

Update - *Just before the publication of this book, I received an email from Summer reporting that she had again spontaneously conceived - naturally!*

Yang Deficiency/Coldness

Features: Whole body is cold, lower back pain and/or knee pain that is relieved by heat, low libido, often lethargic, water retention and a puffy pale bright complexion are common.

Gynecological Features: Cold can cause blockage with blood and bodily fluids creating painful periods with light bleeding known as a cold uterus. Yang Qi deficiency can cause heavy bleeding and copious cervical mucous of watery consistency.
Interpretations: Because of low energy, motivation to exercise is minimal, sometimes encouraging excess weight. Yang deficiency and coldness can often be attached to advanced maternal age and kidney deficiency.

Yang Deficiency/Coldness Example
Barb
- **general info** - Barb was 40 years old and had been trying to conceive for over four years without success. She and her husband were married when she was 35 and began the journey of trying to conceive almost immediately.
- **history** - Medical testing showed that her ovarian reserve was diminished and she was told that her egg quality was most likely poor. Semen analysis showed low motility, morphology and borderline low concentration.
- **presentations** - She had a bright pale complexion, was slightly overweight and complained of

frequently being cold. Her libido was very low. She loved running but had to stop due to pain in her knees. She reported that her menses were very heavy, watery in consistency and contained many large purple clots.

- **pattern(s)** - According to TCM, Barb was very clearly displaying Yang deficient Cold patterns. This was most likely due to a combination of genetics and advanced maternal age.

- **goals** - From a TCM perspective, optimizing her reproductive health and fertility was accomplished by improving her menses, losing weight, improving libido and increasing her subjective body warmth.

- **recommendations & treatment** -
  - Weekly acupuncture appointments and daily Chinese herbal medicine
  - Making sleep a priority
  - Four half-hour sessions of aerobic jogging each week to burn fat
  - Drinking only warm water
  - Focusing on nutrition while drastically limiting raw and cold food intake
  - Creating boundaries on taking work home with her
  - Scheduling regular quality time with friends
  - Cleaning her house and life of all toxic substances
  - Taking high doses of CoQ10

- **outcome** - She reported that her key to being able to stick to the plan was that she wanted to be an example of a healthy mother to her child. This resulted in an overall improvement with her menstrual imbalances, losing 21 pounds, and an increase in sexual interest. Barb became pregnant in just over seven months of TCM treatments. She carried to full term and gave birth to a healthy baby boy.

- **cost** - Approximately $3,800 (included seven

months of weekly acupuncture treatments, daily Chinese herbal medicine and recommended dietary supplements).

Qi Deficiency

Features: Fatigue, poor digestion such as gas and bloating, loose stool, weak immune function, worry, fear and pensiveness.

Gynecological Features: Qi deficiency can cause heavy bleeding and copious cervical mucous of watery consistency. Menstrual cycles may be short with bleeding of heavy volume and watery consistency. Bleeding may also happen outside regular times as in premenstrual spotting.

Interpretations: Fatigue is a common complaint among the Qi deficient. Digestive function can be due to poor food choices and fatigue-based decisions may perpetuate the cycle. Exercise, deep breathing and healthy food choices are often the cure for this mild to moderate state. This can be the early stages of Dampness or Yang deficiency and a good time to make changes before it gets harder to do so.

Qi Deficiency Example
Shannon
- **general info** - Shannon was 35 years-old. Shortly after trying to conceive, she became pregnant. Unfortunately, after eleven weeks, the baby stopped growing and a natural miscarriage followed by a surgical abortion to ensure a full evacuation of the uterus was done. The trauma was immense but she was ready to try again. Fear of another miscarriage was quite powerful and was addressed through the treatment of the Qi of the Kidneys which manages fear and willpower. She had come to traditional Chinese medicine for support as she began her journey of conception

26

again and to be an integral piece in helping produce a healthy pregnancy and carry to term.

- **history** - No medical testing or diagnostics were undertaken. Factor V Laiden (a blood clotting disorder) was in her immediate family so she was considering testing for this as it has implications with blood clotting and possible contributions to miscarriage.

- **presentations** - Shannon had gained a lot of weight since her miscarriage and to her detriment, had an unrelenting work ethic. She did not get enough sleep and had some bad habits such as soda and dairy consumption. She quite clearly had emotional stagnation manifesting as irritability and seemed easily frustrated with others. She showed a number of possible signs of inflammation such as anxiety, restlessness, aversion to heat, cankers, allergies, dry skin, psoriasis and the preference for cold drinks. The Qi deficiency was highlighted by her emotional eating, sweet cravings, ankle swelling, nasal drip, fatigue after eating, difficulty waking in the morning, pensiveness, weight issues and sweating without exertion. She also reported many premenstrual symptoms plaguing her each month.

- **pattern(s)** - According to TCM, Shannon primarily displayed a pattern of Spleen Qi Deficiency. This root pattern was giving rise to the accumulation of both Dampness and Phlegm. The Dampness and Phlegm combined with the moderate Qi Stagnation she also displayed was causing the formation of Heat which was rising to the Heart. The Heart was already experiencing non-free flow due to the emotional toll the second trimester miscarriage had taken on her.

- **goals** - Reducing her weight, allergies, sweet cravings, pensiveness, PMS, menstrual pain, clotting and improving her sleep and cervical mucous.

- **recommendations & treatment -**
  - Weekly acupuncture treatments
  - Stopping the antidepressants she was taking (her decision)
  - Eliminating soda pop and dairy consumption and increasing water intake
  - Incorporating daily femoral massage and nightly foot soaks
  - Finding ways to better manage stress at work
  - Getting more sleep
  - Exercising more
  - Spending more time in nature
  - Avoiding environmental toxins
  - Starting on a whole food homocysteine blend (Vitamin B6, folate, and B12)
  - Adopting a more plant-based whole food diet and reducing starchy carbohydrate intake
  - Getting back in touch with her Christian roots to nourish her spiritual side
- **outcome** - After two months of the above recommendations, Shannon got pregnant. Regular acupuncture continued weekly until 22 weeks when she felt comfortable that all was well with the pregnancy. Her little boy was born healthy and happy a couple of weeks before his due date.
- **cost** - Approximately $2,800 (included 7.5 months of weekly acupuncture treatments and recommended dietary supplements).

Blood Deficiency

<u>Features</u>: Pale complexion and nails, dryness of skin, nose, throat, eyes, hair and nails, scanty menstruation and possible anemia.

<u>Gynecological Features</u>: Light or scanty bleeding that may be pale or diluted with a watery consistency. Cycle is often long as it takes the body more time to mature the

egg and build the uterine lining.

Interpretations: This pattern often accompanies Qi deficiency and is a stage that if left unchecked, may eventually become Yin deficiency. It is most often a result of excessive emotions causing poor digestion which in turn does not produce enough blood.

Blood Deficiency Example
Tina

- **general info** - Tina was a 35 year-old teacher with a very difficult group of students that year. She had been trying to conceive naturally for almost two years. Within this time, she'd had two early miscarriages. She had recently taken some time off work to cope with anxiety and depression. She also admitted to not exercising.
- **history** - Medical testing repeatedly showed iron deficient anemia. Both miscarriages required medications to fully evacuate the pregnancy. Her tubes were clear after a recent hysterosalpingogram (HSG), an x-ray dye test, but they did find and remove two polyps. Tina and her husband were considering IVF but wanted to give TCM a chance first and at the very least, be prepared in body mind and spirit for the IVF.
- **presentations** - Menstrual cycles were usually 35-40 days in length, with very light flow that was pale red and diluted or watery. Her complexion, tongue and nails were very pale and she complained of hair loss, always being tired, dizzy spells, difficulty falling asleep and dull headaches when tired. She had extremely dry skin, poor digestion including, gas, bloating and dry bitty stools and was slightly underweight.
- **pattern(s)** - According to TCM, Tina was presenting with Blood deficiency caused by Spleen deficiency digestive problems, quite likely from a genetic predisposition as her mother is very similar

29

in health history and appearance.

- **goals** - Improving diet and digestion, shortening her cycles and increasing menstrual flow volume, returning colour and moisture back to her skin, supporting her emotionally and helping her sleep better.
- **recommendations & treatment** -
  - Weekly acupuncture treatments and Chinese herbal medicine daily to help build and restore her depleted state.
  - Highly nutritious plant-based whole foods that were mostly cooked to improve digestion. Soups, stews and smoothies were her foundation.
  - Eliminating dairy and increasing water intake.
  - Fish oils, Vitamin D, homocysteine blend (B6, folate, B12) and probiotics were recommended.
  - Consistent yoga practice three times per week
  - One half hour of jogging four times a week
  - Tina also took the remaining five months off of teaching and really took care of herself
- **outcome** - After 20 acupuncture treatments and five months of consistent Chinese herbal medicine administration, Tina's cycles shortened to an average of 30-32 days and bleeding volume increased. She was sleeping better, eating better and felt better overall with more energy and a sense of well-being. She became pregnant again and continued on with the acupuncture and Chinese herbal medicine through the first trimester to help prevent another miscarriage. She had a healthy baby girl.
- **cost** - Approximately $2,900 (included five months of weekly acupuncture treatments, daily Chinese herbal medicine and recommended dietary supplements).

Blood Stasis

Features: Blood Stasis is almost always (aside from trauma) a result of other patterns of disharmony such as Qi stagnation, Coldness, Dampness, Phlegm or Heat. Over time, the condition of Blood Stasis typically leads to Heat and/or Blood deficiency. Common manifestations are fixed stabbing or severe pain, spider veins, dusky complexion and darkening patches of skin.

Gynecological Features: Clotted menstrual bleeding that is brown, purple, or black. Periods will often be light and be severely painful.

Interpretations: Blood Stasis can result from almost any of the other patterns being present over a period of time. If Qi is stagnated, or other blockages ensue due to cold, lack of Yang, Dampness or Heat, eventually blood circulation will be impeded. There is a well-known saying in 'Statements of Fact in TCM' by Bob Flaws that any chronic disease will involve Blood Stasis.

Blood Stasis Example
Samantha
- **general info** - Samantha had recently been through two miscarriages and was not quite ready to get pregnant again. She felt off and wanted to get right. My instincts were that she needed to better manage emotional stress, improve blood circulation and have her heart healed. Ultimately she needed a break from her in-laws but that wasn't possible so we utilized Chinese medicine to help her adjust to her circumstances.
- **history** - Her doctors had told her she couldn't get any testing done as she had not had three losses and that it was likely an egg quality issue. Basic fertility testing had never been done. Even if diagnostic testing had taken place, there is little treatment for recurrent loss.

31

- **presentations** - Fear and frustration trumped all else with Samantha. Sleep was very light and plagued with night sweats. She suffered from intense pelvic pain during sex and on the first two days of her period. Both back and neck pain were also quite severe. She had spider veins and darkening patches of skin particularly around her armpits and near skin folds. Her tongue was purple and dusky in colour and her cervical mucous was scant.
- **pattern(s)** - According to TCM, she was clearly presenting both Blood Stasis and Qi Stagnation, so our primary principles of treatment were to restore optimal blood circulation and soothe emotional blockage.
- **goals** - Soothing emotions and managing stress to reduce the chances of miscarriage and aid in carrying pregnancy to term. Instilling more peace of mind and stress reduction surrounding circumstances in her life, helping her mind and body heal and get strong enough to conquer her fear and feel ready to conceive again, improving sleep, reducing pelvic pain, eliminating night sweats, reducing back pain and neck tension and increasing cervical mucous.
- **recommendations & treatment** -
  - Weekly acupuncture treatments and Chinese herbal medicine daily
  - A dietary cleanse for one month
  - With everything that was going on in her life that was out of her control, I strongly suggested doing some work with our Integrated Professional Life Coach, Thomas Kevin Dolan
  - Supplements including Vitamin D, fish oils, CoQ10, and a homocysteine blend (Vitamin B6, folate, B12)
  - Eliminating soda pop, dairy and gluten
  - Avoiding toxins that are known endocrine

    disruptors
- Moderate exercise
- Nurturing her spirit
- Self-administering castor oil packs and femoral massage in her follicular phase (cycle day 1 to ovulation) to help optimize blood circulation to reproductive organs

- **outcome** - From my experience, Blood Stasis and Qi Stagnation are two patterns that respond quite quickly to treatment with acupuncture and Chinese herbal medicine. When treatment restores overall smooth flow to both Qi and Blood, these are the types of stories I receive:

"When I met Spence, he listened to my thoughts, fears and concerns. It was nice to be able to tell someone everything I had kept inside for so long. Spence was extremely kind and compassionate, he seemed to understand exactly what I was feeling and going through. I left his office feeling hopeful, and went home feeling positive. My husband seemed relieved and somewhat excited to see me so happy. I no longer felt alone. I felt like someone was working with me toward a common goal and was going to help me. It was a good feeling. It has now been a little under two months since I first met Spence. In this time, I have been receiving acupuncture sessions and taking Chinese herbs at Spence's recommendation. I have cut sugar, gluten and dairy from my diet completely. I have never felt better. I can't really explain what has started to bring my sense of self-back. I can't even explain what made me awaken and realize that I needed to stand still, surrender and embrace what was happening to me. I needed to live in the moment enjoying what I have, in this moment. As I sit here writing this, I feel a smile on my face, and warmth in my heart that I have not felt for a long time. No, I am not pregnant, not yet anyway, but I am no

longer afraid to try again. What I have realized in this short time is that I matter, and for so long I had forgotten that. I wish I had walked into Spence's office a year ago, but it's never too late for anything. I truly believe that Spence has made a difference in my life. Whether it's the Acupuncture, the herbs or my healthy diet; my body, mind and spirit has started to find its way back to me. I feel light-hearted, happier and hopeful. My husband has noticed a drastic difference in my mood, my body language and my overall presence. I am very grateful to Spence; his guidance and kindness has truly made a difference in my life."

The cycle after she wrote this, Samantha became pregnant again. She continued with weekly acupuncture treatments and daily Chinese herbal medicine through her first trimester. This time she carried to term with no complications.

- **cost** - Approximately $3,000 (included 5.5 months of weekly acupuncture treatments, daily Chinese herbal medicine and recommended dietary supplements - including first trimester of pregnancy).

Qi Stagnation

"Holding onto Anger is like drinking poison and expecting the other person to die." ~Buddha

Features: Qi stagnation, most typically of the liver, has its causative root in the deregulation of emotions. Common manifestations are feeling emotionally stuck, irritable, angry, impatient, frustrated, unfulfilled and stressed out.

Gynecological Features: Length of menstrual cycle will often be irregular--sometimes late, sometimes early with bleeding that starts and stops. Mild to moderate pain before and during the period is common. PMS signs and symptoms such as moodiness, breast tenderness, nausea and bloating are prominent.

Interpretations: If a person feels stuck, unfulfilled, not in control of their emotions, stressed out, overwhelmed and full of anxiety, then they likely have Qi stagnation. One might say that to some degree, this is almost every adult on earth and they are right. Management of this pattern is a part of every treatment plan I create. It should be highlighted that there are many degrees and severities of this pattern.

Qi Stagnation Example
Charlotte

- **general info** - Already very frustrated and impatient, 33 year-old lawyer Charlotte had been trying to conceive for seven months so inducing a greater state of inner peace was my ultimate goal for her. Being calm does not mean getting less done; it is just an adjustment of attitude while completing tasks. She was a very strong lady who knew what she wanted and was ready to put the plans into action to accomplish her goals. We went through exactly what the next three months would look like so that I could be Charlotte's accountability partner each week when we met.
- **history** - No medical testing had been done to date except basic blood work such as thyroid and complete blood count, which was all normal. I suggested an HSG to check if her tubes were clear.
- **presentations** - In addition to being a very Type 'A' (i.e., supercharged, impatient, restless and over-exercising), her bowel movements alternated from loose to constipated and felt unfinished. She had sleep issues, partook in emotional eating, experienced headaches, cold hands and feet, neck tension, sighing, night sweats, low libido, acne, difficulty waking in morning, gas and bloating,

was slightly overweight and craved sweets. She had only three days of menstrual flow that was clotted and moderately painful with many prominent premenstrual symptoms.

- **pattern(s)** - According to TCM, she presented with textbook Qi Stagnation. This also caused concurrent patterns such as mild Blood Stasis, depressive Heat rising to her Heart and Qi deficiency which resulted in some Dampness accumulation.

- **goals** - To calm her spirit and reduce restlessness, irritability and impatience. I also wanted to relieve her back pain, increase menstrual blood flow, reduce clotting and PMS, improve her sleep, regulate bowel movements, reduce headaches, neck tension and sighing, improve her digestion and encourage weight loss.

- **recommendations & treatment** -
    - Weekly acupuncture treatments and Chinese herbal medicine daily
    - Changing her thinking about down time being boring and unproductive. The word 'opening' which is what acupuncture does, was brought up a lot. She really resonated with the concept of conception being about reception, not accomplishment. It is often a challenge to explain to people how TCM will benefit them in a language they understand. Since she was a litigator, I used the language of negotiation (i.e., I will allow two Yin yoga classes each week if she gave up two of her three spin classes). We did this with various dietary concepts and lifestyle habits as well. It was quite incredible how involved she was in the creation of her plan and when negotiations were done, she was passionately committed and excited. It was inspiring to see.
    - Understanding when ovulation was occurring through self-monitoring

- **outcome** - The transformations I was fortunate
  enough to witness with this woman paid off
  quickly. After only two months of deep
  commitment to our plan, she became pregnant and
  nine months later gave birth to a healthy little girl.
  She continued with acupuncture through the first
  and most of the second trimester of pregnancy as
  there was much spotting and lots of debilitating
  nausea, then powerful headaches throughout the
  first few weeks of the second trimester. It is cases
  like these that I cherish deeply. When I get to
  watch someone's whole life shift toward wellness,
  I know the effects of our time together will have
  positive implications on her health and well-being
  forever.
- **cost** - Approximately $2500 (included six months
  of weekly acupuncture treatments, recommended
  dietary supplements, and two months of pre-
  pregnancy daily Chinese herbal medicine).

In Step Three, we will go into the importance of diet in
curing these conditions and which foods will be beneficial
and what to avoid.

Integration

I respect western medicine; it has given us so much. I
have seen assisted reproductive technologies such as In
Vitro Fertilization (IVF) help women and couples have
children that otherwise would not have been able to; for
example, with blocked fallopian tubes. It is a wonderful
technology that can help improve any woman or couples'
chances of conception. Without western medicine,
premature babies would rarely survive, penicillin would
not have saved millions of lives and many more women
would still be dying in childbirth. It is my belief that both
western and eastern medicine have something to
contribute and when used together, can have greater
results. In fact, I believe we live in a time where the

integration of different styles of medicine and healing are producing a massive leap in the evolution of human health.

But the philosophies do vary quite drastically.

Reductionism (the belief that any complex system is nothing more than the sum of its parts) is the foundation of western medical practice. Western practice uses randomized controlled research and statistics to explain the human body and to categorize people. Traditional Chinese Medicine takes into account the whole individualized picture and is aptly referred to as (w)holistic (the belief that the whole is greater than the sum of its parts).

From a western medical perspective, the top three diagnosis women come to me with are:

Unexplained
There is no such thing as unexplained infertility in Chinese Medicine. Unexplained just means we have to look harder and get to the root of things. It takes commitment and perseverance but there is an explanation and together we will find it and fix it. Quite often this has an emotional component and that is something that is very hard to measure but often not hard to fix.

Male Factor
We'll talk more about this in Step Ten, but in short, the man is just as responsible for healthy conception as the woman. Because a woman carries the baby and the importance of egg quality dominates western medical thinking, a lot of the blame for infertility is often placed on her when in fact the man plays a vital role in conception. His diet and lifestyle are just as important to his sperm quality as a woman's is to her eggs. The Chinese have a beautiful term for the constitution of an unborn child--"pre-heaven essence" and the future father

38

of a child contributes exactly half of this poetic terminology.

Advanced Maternal Age (AMA)
Like unexplained infertility, this is a bit of a catch-all phrase that can be specified and often overcome with some digging and dedication. While it may be easier to get pregnant in your twenties, as long as a woman is still menstruating there is potential to bear children.

By contrast, the six causes of infertility and any other disease in the body according to Chinese Medicine are:

> External Evils: *From a modern perspective this would include bacteria, viruses, medications, environmental toxins and/or smoking, as well as some mental disorders.*

> Overwork: *Since age is a considerable factor in infertility these days, ask yourself if you are putting financial certainty before having a child. If you are working too hard, is there even room for a baby? If a baby is your priority, then it is important to live your life in a way that is conducive to the welcoming of this priority. Career or financial advancement must take a back seat, or at the very least share the spotlight.*

> Diet: *We will go into more detail about finding what is right for you in the step on diet but in short, lots of colorful food provides the required nutrition for fertility and healthy pregnancy, and portions need to be controlled.*

> Emotions: *Stress creates disease and comes in many disguises from sadness and anger to loneliness and anxiety. We will talk more about this throughout the book because its impact is huge. Remember to check in with yourself*

*throughout the day and take a deep breath to see
where you're at. Healthy mind, healthy body.*

Activity Level: *Too much or too little can be
detrimental so find what's right for you. If you're
at a desk all day, go for a 20-minute walk or
incorporate some stretches in your day. And if you
train every day and participate in a triathlon every
three months, maybe slow down a little. It's all
about finding balance.*

Trauma: *Your body is both immensely strong and a
delicate balance. Trauma can be interpreted as
STI's, a D&C procedure (surgical procedure used
to clean the uterus of the products of conception
due to a non-viable pregnancy or abortion),
injuries sustained from sporting accidents
(particularly for men), surgery or a car accident
that has thrown off pelvic structure. There are
corrections for these traumas though, so don't feel
like there is nothing you can do or it's out of your
hands.*

As far as fertility is concerned, there are both obvious and
some not-so-obvious adaptations a person can make to
their lives in order to get a handle on these causes, putting
the patient much more in a proactive role rather than
feeling helpless. And that brings me to our next topic:
what can you do? Set some goals.

What does a course of TCM treatment involve?

Since the most important paradigm of TCM is the
individualization of treatment, courses of action will vary
from person to person to meet their specific needs. The
two primary tools are Acupuncture and Chinese herbal
medicine. They may be used separately or in combination,
depending on the requirements of the patient and
determined by the doctor.

Acupuncture is usually administered one to two times per week, and Chinese herbal medicine is taken daily via pills or teas. Consistency and commitment are key for treatment to be effective.

Here are some examples of conditions I see and possible accompanying treatment plans:

- **Polycystic Ovary Syndrome (PCOS)** is determined by the presence of multiple cysts on the ovaries, excess androgen levels (male hormones), irregular ovulation and menstrual cycles, and insulin resistance . PCOS is a condition that often requires six to twelve months of acupuncture and herbal medicine to restore hormonal balance and regular ovulation. Ideally we like to see three healthy menstrual cycles before trying to conceive and falling pregnant. Due to miscarriage rates being higher in this patient population, TCM treatment continues through the first trimester of pregnancy.
- **Unexplained infertility** often responds very favorably with two to three months of TCM treatments. This is a diagnosis common in women in their early 30's. If there are no other confounding conditions, women with unexplained infertility very often fall pregnant within six months of starting TCM.
- Women and couples that have decided to go through **In Vitro Fertilization (IVF)** can increase their chances of success and decrease the associated stress levels by incorporating TCM into the weeks and months prior to the IVF treatment. Our goal for any woman is to have at least nine acupuncture treatments in the 2.5 to 3 months before embryo transfer. Depending on the presenting reproductive health conditions, more time and more treatment before starting the IVF may be recommended (this often includes the

husband if male factor infertility is present). In the 2-4 weeks before embryo transfer, Chinese herbal medicine is stopped (unless it is a special case) and acupuncture is increased in frequency to twice per week. Our treatment goals at this time are to regulate emotions, reduce stress and promote blood circulation through the reproductive organs to improve ovarian and uterine response to IVF medications. Then two acupuncture treatments are administered on site at the IVF clinic immediately before and after embryo transfer. Following transfer, acupuncture treatments are again recommended once a week until the end of the first trimester to ensure pregnancy is stable, nausea is managed and your body is supported during the hormonal changes that are occurring.

- **Stress and anxiety** can show drastic improvements in only one to two months of consistent acupuncture and lifestyle modifications.
- **Recurrent pregnancy loss (RPL)** is largely about providing emotional support, the cultivation of willpower and the management of fear, as well as improving circulation issues that could be impeding healthy pregnancies. I often recommend at least two to three months without trying to conceive after a miscarriage, even if the body and menstrual cycle have bounced back to a state of health and regularity. For most women, this is time is well spent healing the heart and preparing the body for another pregnancy. Then again when pregnant, treatment continues throughout the first trimester and often much further or the whole pregnancy in its entirety, mostly due to the request of the mother-to-be. It should also be noted that sperm may be playing a role in recurrent loss, so treating the male partner is also important.
- **Male factor infertility** is more cut and dry. With many men, there are very few health signs and symptoms to monitor (in comparison to a woman

and menstrual cycle characteristics) and determine treatment benefits, so we assume that sperm quality is being affected with the proper consistent administration of acupuncture, Chinese herbal medicine and lifestyle recommendations. Twelve acupuncture treatments within a six to twelve week period is considered one course of treatment, and often two courses of treatment are required to see improvement.

- **Thyroid conditions** such as hypothyroidism or require dedication and in my experience at least six months of TCM, supplements and lifestyle changes to ensure balance optimal for conception.
- **Advanced Maternal Age (AMA)** and **Diminished Ovarian Reserve (DOR)** require acupuncture one to two times per week until pregnancy is confirmed, then continues throughout much of the first two trimesters. Chinese herbal medicine is absolutely necessary in these cases. This treatment often requires six to twelve months to begin to display effect. If assisted reproductive technologies such as IVF with PGD (Preimplantation Genetic Diagnosis) are being considered, TCM offers support and optimization for success. I counsel this patient population not to wait very long before making this choice, as it is well known that age is the single most important determining factor in IVF success. Time is of the essence.
- Our primary goal with **Endometriosis** is to reduce pain which in my experience TCM is extremely effective for. Our secondary goals are to improve fertility, balance hormone levels and reduce inflammation surrounding the ovaries and uterus. Acupuncture is recommended once to twice per week and Chinese herbal medicine is taken daily until noticeable changes have been observed. It may be necessary to adjust frequency of the acupuncture sessions to address a certain time and

need during the menstrual cycle. In some cases, symptoms get worse around ovulation and continue to increase in intensity until menstruation, therefore more frequent treatment during this time may be indicated. In other cases, the pain is felt only with menstruation, while others experience pain throughout their cycle. Our goal is to see three menstrual cycles with minimal or complete absence of pain. This indicates to us that levels of inflammation have decreased and hormone levels are returning to a more healthy balance.

- **Pregnancy-related conditions** such as nausea and pain, as well as turning breech babies and preparing for labour, are all strong suits of TCM. Pain is usually addressed with frequent acupuncture treatments until relief is obtained. Nausea is most often only an affliction of the first trimester, and depending on severity, one to three acupuncture treatments per week may be necessary. Moxibustion to turn breech babies is best done between the 33rd and 36th week, and preparing for labour involves the administration of acupuncture once per week from week 36-40.

Story
Suzanne W.

"I was 36.5 when my husband and I decided to start a family and within three months, I was pregnant. I had an easy pregnancy and an easy birth and we loved being parents so two years later, we started trying for our second. Since we'd had such an easy time with our first daughter, we didn't think it would be a problem, but after six months of trying with no luck, we decided to seek help. Doctors told me that I essentially had no eggs left and that my FSH levels were 16-20. I was told that I had a 4% chance at best, possibly 8% with the highest dose of fertility drugs and that my best bet was to go to the U.S.

for an egg donation. The thought of buying an egg wasn't what I wanted but I had to consider my husband.

We were shocked and devastated. We wondered how this was possible, when we'd had a daughter so easily two years before. I kept the entire ordeal to myself, with the exception of my mom. I didn't want to hear any unsolicited advice or sympathy from people.

After hormone shots and a failed IUI attempt, we decided we would try a round of IVF and if it didn't work we would decide the next steps, probably to stop trying and try to be happy with one child, but I know we would have been very disappointed. We went through the hormone shots again and they thought they may be able to retrieve three eggs but after harvest, we only had one viable egg. I was beyond disappointed – the women in recovery next to me had twelve eggs! That Friday we went home with little hope. They would give us updates to see if the embryo would multiply. Miraculously, it did! It was amazing and on Monday we went back to have it implanted. Just before my 40th birthday in March, we were told we were pregnant.

I did acupuncture with Dr. Pentland once a week leading up to the IVF implantation. The day of implantation, I had before and after treatment, then continued until I was pregnant and throughout the pregnancy up to about 6 months. The sessions left me feeling peaceful, relaxed and positive.

I was monitored quite regularly since the doctors were worried about miscarriage and high blood pressure and I truly believe that the acupuncture, relaxation and positive energy from Spence were a big reason the IVF worked and I carried to term a healthy baby girl. Listening to the tapes and imagining the egg and uterus was amazing. I don't usually go for non-traditional, non-western medicine but I know this is what kept me relaxed.

45

Doctors said once a year they get the "amazing" result and we were the couple. I was the only woman with a less than 5% chance that had one egg on the first try that was successful.

Today we have two daughters, Katherine who is four and a half, and miracle baby Hannah who is a year and a half now. We are done and we are so happy. Being a parent is the most rewarding job in the world and also the hardest. It teaches you unconditional love, selflessness and patience."

Chapter Task:

List three things you learned about TCM:

1. _____

2. _____

3. _____

For reference, list *your* top 2 or 3 TCM patterns (i.e., Heat, Qi Stagnation, Dampness, etc.)

1 ._____

2. _____

3. _____

Write down any questions you still have about TCM:

_____

_____

_____

_____

_____

Bring these questions to your Doctor of TCM.

<u>Step Two</u>

Goal Setting:

Getting from point A to point B by breaking down what needs to be done

"Change is never a matter of ability, it is always a matter of motivation born from a compelling 'why'. Once you are clear on your 'why' setting goals is the first step in turning the invisible into the visible." ~Tony Robbins

The goal of anyone experiencing infertility is to have a child. When times are trying, and you are adapting your lifestyle in what might be challenging ways, that is the goal that needs to be kept in mind. Sometimes when you've been trying for a while, this ultimate goal can seem frustratingly unreachable so breaking it down into more manageable steps is key. That's what we're going to talk about in this section.

It is my belief that the most important step in achieving anything is the process of goal setting. Without a target, how can one hit it? With clear goals and vision, each choice you make throughout each day can be evaluated by asking yourself, is this choice bringing me closer to my dream?

As a doctor, I determine my goals for treatment from the initial intake forms and the first appointment. By diagnosing the prominent signs and symptoms I feel are important to work on, combined with our joint decisions about larger aspects of life and your family vision, we provide the framework for setting goals. These goals become a guide to ensure we are staying on the path that we have created together.

Once your goals are clear and you are doing everything in your power to obtain them, it is time to surrender. Not everyone is ready to hear this and it can be tough to relinquish control, but having faith in your body is of paramount importance. Patience is one of the primary attributes of a good parent and you might want to think of this time as a dress rehearsal for what's to come.

While each person's path to fertility will vary, I have found that after a decade of working with couples trying to conceive that the following four steps can be a recipe for success:

1. Take care of yourself (set those goals).
2. Do your best to surrender and accept your circumstances.
3. Have faith that your dreams will come true.
4. Persevere.

Breaking down your goals into obtainable and sustainable steps and sticking with them for enough time to allow the magic of the compound effect to manifest is the key to success. When setting goals, remember the wise words of Jim Collins (author of 'Good to Great'): "*If you have more than three priorities, you don't have any.*" Figure out what is most necessary for you to do to accomplish your goals, forget about everything else and keep it simple.

Here are some examples of possible goals for specific reproductive health conditions (the use of TCM should be assumed with each condition presented):

Polycystic Ovary Syndrome (PCOS):
With PCOS, ideally, our main goal is to see three healthy regular menstrual cycles before trying to conceive. When the recommended plan and lifestyle changes below are

deeply committed to, three healthy regular menstrual cycles and pregnancy can be achieved for some within a 6-12 month TCM treatment period. PCOS is most often multifactorial and the clinical picture can vary drastically from woman to woman. Irregular ovulation, excess androgens (male hormones), and issues with insulin resistance or blood sugar balance are the current diagnostic triad of PCOS (a woman does not have to present with cystic ovaries to receive this diagnosis). Therefore, the goals of a woman with PCOS may look something like this:

- Hormonal balance - A myriad of hormonal storms are often associated with PCOS. A thorough endocrine evaluation is recommended to properly guide treatment (thyroid, adrenals, ovarian, pituitary, pancreatic, etc.).
- Diet - Low carbohydrate/sugar, high fiber, whole foods and proteins. The glycemic load must be reduced when insulin resistance and blood sugar imbalance is present. Reduction of portions if necessary.
- Inositol (Vitamin B8) - May aid in the balancing of androgens and estrogens, stabilize mood and make cells more sensitive to insulin. For more information, see Step Five.
- Exercise - especially if overweight, both aerobic fat burning and weight training are essential to success in management of PCOS. Regular weight training is very effective in the regulation of blood sugar.
- Electro-acupuncture (acupuncture with the addition of small electrodes on needles to enhance stimulation) - Acupuncture administered once per week for an average of 15-20 weeks helps restore regular ovulation in many women. A study recently published in the journal, Acta Diabetologia, showed that acupuncture decreased insulin resistance (Benrick, 2014).

51

"There is an immeasurable distance between late and too late." ~Og Mandino

Advanced Maternal Age (AMA):
The primary goal with AMA is to optimize the quality of the remaining eggs, ovarian and uterine environment, and reproductive essence. Simply put, eliminating everything we know that causes aging is required. Most people understand what not to do if the desire is to look radiant and keep skin looking young. Fertility is not that different, as your skin, similarly to fertility, is a manifestation of your overall health and well-being. It should also be emphasized that just because you are of advanced maternal age, it doesn't mean that you will not have the family you dream of. The path may just require a little more work on your part. In this age group (>38), if IVF is being considered, preimplantation genetic diagnosis (PGD) is a new advancement that may play a key role in success. It may be slightly cost prohibitive at the time of this publication, but I strongly encourage learning more about this comprehensive chromosomal screening to see if it is the right fit for you. A sample goal list for women of advanced maternal age would be something like this:

- Exercise - To ensure good circulation, regular cardio is a must. This also helps with stress.
- Sleep - The importance of sleep cannot be overstated. This is when the body gets a chance to regenerate and nourish itself. Make getting enough quality sleep a priority.
- Reducing workload - When we are not 25 but want our body to act this way, we must give ourselves the time required to nurture oneself, to slow down and conserve vital energy and focus for reproduction.
- Nutrition - Special attention needs to be given to eating highly nutritious foods to ensure that the body is getting more than it requires. For more

information see Step Five.

- CoQ10 - Preliminary evidence shows CoQ10 may have an effect on improving egg quality. For more information see Step Five.

Diminished Ovarian Reserve (DOR) / High FSH / Low AMH / Low AFC:

Often, but not always associated with age, diminished ovarian reserve, i.e., low AFC (antral follicle count), high FSH (follicle stimulating hormone) and low AMH (antimullerian hormone) are all important test results which show a woman may be close to the end of her reproductive years and that egg quality may not be what it once was. This is a very challenging time for women as the clock begins ticking more loudly and many IVF centres may not even accept them as patients. At this point, a woman's chances of conceiving naturally may be better (with the aid of TCM and acupuncture, supplements and lifestyle changes) than with IVF or other assisted reproductive technologies (ART). There is still hope, and it is important that you do not turn against yourself with emotions of regret, anger and resentment. This is a time more than ever when you must put trust in your body and do all you can to restore balance and deep holistic health to your life. The following suggestions are important if you have received this diagnosis:

- Chinese herbal medicine - This is likely one of the most powerful tools that exists when attempting to improve their reproductive potential when faced with any or all of these diagnosis. Six to twelve months of administration is recommended.
- Anti-inflammatory diet - Inflammation could very well be contributing to this diminished reproductive essence and hormonal imbalance. Understand what foods should be avoided. *Refer to the notes on inflammatory foods in the chapter on diet for more information. Consider a cleanse to kick start this learning process. I recommend

Mediclear from Thorne Research to my patients.

- <u>Assisted reproductive technology</u> - Especially if age is a factor, this is a diagnosis where I encourage considering IVF sooner than later, if it is an option. As stated above, if IVF is being considered, preimplantation genetic diagnosis (PGD) is a new advancement that may play a key role in success.

- <u>Qigong</u> - An ancient Chinese form of exercise involving soft movement and meditative breathing. Used for the cultivation of deep health, longevity. This is one of the few ways the Chinese believe one can reverse diminishing reproductive essence.

- <u>Perseverance</u> - The single most important quality one can possess when faced with odds such as this. Do not give up.

NOTE: *DHEA (Dehydroepiandrosterone) supplementation in diminished ovarian reserve (DOR) has been reported to improve pregnancy chances with DOR, and is now utilized by approximately one third of all IVF centers worldwide. Increasing DHEA utilization and publication of a first prospectively randomized trial warranted a systematic review. Current best available evidence suggests that DHEA improves ovarian function, increases pregnancy chances and, by reducing aneuploidy (abnormal chromosomal make up), lowers miscarriage rates. DHEA over time also appears to objectively improve ovarian reserve. Recent animal data support androgens (male hormones) in promoting preantral follicle growth ('sleeping follicles') and reduction in follicle atresia (death). Improvement of egg/embryo quality with DHEA supplementation potentially suggests a new concept of ovarian aging, where **ovarian environments**, but not eggs themselves, age. DHEA may, thus, represent a first agents beneficially affecting aging ovarian environments (Gleicher, 2011). Other agents (foods, supplements, medications, lifestyle interventions) can be expected to show improvement of aging **ovarian***

environments*. This is precisely what I (and countless colleagues) have always believed that Traditional Chinese Medicine was accomplishing, improving the 'whole' reproductive environment. I look forward to the day science catches up and shows that Chinese herbs and acupuncture have been improving ovarian environments (egg quality) all along!*

Unexplained Infertility:
With unexplained fertility, there are many possibilities. I would say the first goal is to determine where your particular challenges lay. The good news is that by enlisting a doctor of TCM, you have taken the first step.

In my experience, this is a condition that responds favorably and quickly with TCM. Together we will find out what is standing between you and a baby. One of the common themes I see with unexplained fertility is emotional. So you might want to set the goal of discovering what your emotions are and if they are negative, what you can do to overcome them. Your goal list might look something like this:

- Meditation - Check out the local meditation centres (often Buddhist), read up on the subject and ultimately take 10 minutes a day (or more if you can spare it) of quiet time to sit alone with your thoughts in an attempt to cultivate more peace. This is a practice so have patience with yourself.
- Fun - Are you getting enough? When I asked Martha, an absolutely fabulous and vibrant 88 year-old woman in my Qigong class, what is her most profound pearl of wisdom after living such a long life, she responded by saying; 'Don't take life too seriously.' Sometimes it's that simple.
- Yoga - Research classes and times that are convenient. In Vancouver where I live, there are more yoga studios than Starbucks. First time drop-

ins are usually free, so take some time to find a style and place that you feel is a fit for you.

- Coaching or Counselling - Keep a regular appointment with someone you respect and trust that can guide you through this journey.
- Give back - Find ways to contribute to your community. Step outside yourself and your circumstance. Volunteer.
  "It is one of the most beautiful compensations of life that no person can sincerely try to help another without helping themself." ~Ralph Waldo Emerson
- Journal - Buy a beautiful journal and fill it with all of your thoughts. This is a great way to discover what's going on for you. It is also a great way to dispose of the garbage and self-defeat floating in your mind.

Thin Uterine Lining:
One of the major causes of infertility and IVF failure is a thin uterine lining and inadequate blood flow to the uterus. Treatment to increase blood flow is essential to improving fertility and reducing chances of miscarriage. It should be noted that stress, lack of exercise, not enough rest, lack of joy and certain foods can inhibit blood flow to the uterus and ovaries. The following are effective treatments for a thin uterine lining.

- Acupuncture - Proven effective via observation with Doppler ultrasound by researchers from Sweden (Stener-Victorin, 1996 & 2003) for increasing blood flow to the reproductive organs. In my clinical experience, acupuncture is extremely effective for the management of thin uterine lining.
- Diet - Avoid sour food when bleeding (yogurt, vinegar, pickles, grapefruit, currants, green apples, etc.) Consume more blood invigorating foods when bleeding (fish, ginger, cinnamon, turmeric).

Post menstruation, eat blood nourishing foods (eggs, carrots, spinach, dates, goji berries).

- Castor Oil packs - Recommended at night in conjunction with foot soaks (see Step Eight).
- Sleep - You need a minimum of seven restful hours of sleep to recharge your body and allow for optimal repair and growth to take place.
- Exercise - Mild cardio, yoga and brisk walking will help with optimal blood circulation.
- Vitamin D & Fish oils - Both of these supplements are important when a woman's lining is thin. For more information, refer to Step Five.

Endometriosis:
In the case of Endometriosis, our primary goals (to enhance fertility) are balancing hormone levels and reducing inflammation surrounding the ovaries and uterus, as well as reducing pain. To date, exact mechanisms underlying Endometriosis are still up for debate. There is still much one can do to manage pain and create a healthier environment for the reproductive organs.

- Visceral manipulation - A properly trained massage therapist may be able to aid in the softening or healing of pelvic adhesions caused by Endometriosis.
- Indole 3 Carbinol, Magnesium, & N-Acetylcysteine - These as well as other supplements may help the body better manage this condition via hormone regulation, nourishing deficiencies, reducing pain, and limiting or reducing the growth of Endometriosis. See Step Five for more information.
- Acupuncture & Chinese herbal medicine - Extremely effective for the management of menstrual pain associated with Endometriosis.
- Brussels sprouts - Liver health is required to properly convert and eliminate proliferative estrogen, which can be high in women with

Endometriosis. Including cruciferous vegetables in your diet such as broccoli, Brussels sprouts, cabbage, collards, cauliflower, kale and turnips will aid liver with this important task.

- Avoid toxins - Many toxins in our environment are known to disrupt hormonal balance and are major contributors to conditions such as Endometriosis. You can read more about this topic in Step Seven.

According to the collaborative on health and the environment and conditions database, PCB's and their cousin PCDD (dioxins) are linked to Endometriosis. The most common sources of human contact are through beef and dairy consumption. It is likely why we have seen massive improvements in women with Endometriosis when they completely eliminate dairy from their diets.

Pelvic Pain (Vulvodynia):
In addition to infertility, women with pelvic pain can lose interest in sex extremely quickly. It is important to understand when your fertile time is. The body naturally adjusts to be more accommodating to sex during your fertile times. In the days leading up to ovulation, cervical fluid should increase helping with lubrication, and the cervix should soften and retract upwards into the vagina creating an environment that is comfortable for penetration. If the pain is unbearable, sex should be kept exclusively to this time of your cycle. Developing relaxation techniques (deep breathing, visualization) prior to and during sexual activity will also help.

- Counselling - If there is a past event that may be contributing to this, it is essential that it be addressed.
- Feeling fertile - Know when you are fertile (prior to ovulation), as sex is most often much more comfortable at this time of the menstrual cycle.
- Avoid cold drinks and cold food - May increase

cytokine activity, which increases pain response and intensity.
- Physiotherapy - Assessment and treatment is sometimes quite useful. Find a professional who specializes in the pelvic floor.
- Muscle relaxation - Learn to relax your muscles, both the pelvic floor as well as those that carry tension from everyday life such as your shoulders, hips and jaw.

Recurrent Pregnancy Loss:

"I know God will not give me anything I can't handle. I just wish that He didn't trust me so much."
~Mother Teresa

With women that have suffered from pregnancy loss, addressing the needs of the spirit is always a primary principle of treatment. The emotions of sadness and anger that accompany this loss and the fear attached to trying again, sometimes seem insurmountable. Medical causes for the loss must also be understood when possible, then addressed if treatment exists. Regulation of the immune system and ensuring proper blood circulation are imperative in the treatment protocol. TCM is a very effective treatment option for soothing emotions, balancing hormones, promoting blood circulation and regulation of the immune system—all important aspects that may be involved in a large percentage of miscarriages. There is also evidence that if IVF is being considered, preimplantation genetic diagnosis (PGD) is a new advancement that may play a key role in preventing miscarriage. Though costly, I encourage learning more about this chromosomal screening technology to see if it is right for you. Other recommendations are:

- Counselling/coaching - Counselling to help deal with the pain associated with the loss and coaching to help you get back on your feet, reduce fear and once again move toward your goal.

- Yoga - Great for the body mind and spirit. Helps improve posture and eliminate any structural issues that may be contributing to improper physical function of reproductive organs.
- Coffee and alcohol - Eliminate. These have both been associated with increased risk of elevated homocysteine levels and miscarriage.
- Homocysteine - Elevated homocysteine levels* may contribute to miscarriage. Adding supplements and eating foods high in B6, B9 (folic acid - specifically 5-MTHF), and B12 help regulate homocysteine.
- Avoid stress - Especially when pregnant, do everything in your power to avoid stress. Stress reduces nutrition and blood flow to the developing embryo.

Homocysteine: increased homocysteine levels are associated with inflammation of blood vessels and the reduction of blood flow to surrounding tissues (i.e., uterus).

Pregnancy Loss. Unburden your Heart.
By Dr. Erin Flynn

Trying to get pregnant after a miscarriage is an emotional journey. If a woman has suffered several miscarriages, the journey has taken a toll on both her body and her spirit. Often, questions of why and how are being asked – is it because of my egg quality? Is there a genetic incompatibility? Is there something wrong with my uterus? What about immunological or blood clotting factors? Endocrine or thyroid reasons? Am I really "unexplainable"?

As Chinese Medicine doctors, we are asking the same questions. But the wording and the ideas we use are a little different – how nourished is your Kidney Yin? How is your Kidney Yang functioning? What does your constitution indicate about your Jing and your Qi? What is the condition of your Blood – are there any signs of stagnation, deficiency, or heat? Are there any indications of dampness or phlegm, and if so are there also heat signs? What is happening at a more holistic level with your sleep, digestion, thirst, energy, body temperature? Any aches and pains?

And there is one more very important factor which also needs to be assessed. It is sometimes overlooked - how is your Heart handling the ups and the downs of your pregnancies and your losses? Have you put up an emotional shield of self-defence so that you do not feel the pain? Do tears fall frequently and uncontrollably? How is your emotional stability during the day, and are you having any bad dreams? Have you acknowledged and grieved for your loss? Have you accepted the experience that you've had, and are you open and ready to invite a new experience in? Are you able to forgive yourself? Can you surrender to the process?

In biomedicine, we talk about the HPO Axis (the Hypothalamus – Pituitary – Ovarian Axis). This refers to

A study of 238 women undergoing IVF treatment showed those who received acupuncture had significantly less first trimester miscarriages when compared to the women that did not receive acupuncture (Khorram, 2012).

the hormonal interconnection between the brain and the reproductive organs. Stress, anxiety and strong emotions are known to disrupt this cycle, often manifesting as menstrual and fertility difficulties. This is the Mind-Body connection.

In Chinese Medicine, we talk about the communication between the Heart and the Kidneys as being similar to the HPO Axis. Let's face it – miscarriage is a heart-breaking experience. And your Heart needs to heal from it so that healthy, fertile communication with your Kidneys can resume. Emotional numbness, uncontrollable crying, depression and nightmares can be indicators of a Heart energy not in balance.

Sometimes the energy of the Heart can be brought back into balance by simply acknowledging how sad it is to lose a pregnancy, and by having a good cry with someone you trust. Spending time in nature where the energy of life surrounds you can be therapeutic. Sometimes we can use certain acupuncture points on the Heart, Pericardium and Liver meridians to help restore and ground Heart energy. There are Chinese Herbal Formulas we can use to help nourish and clear the Heart. And some women will really benefit from seeing a Therapist or Clinical Counsellor who has experience working with reproductive health related challenges.

So as you are trying to make sense of your journey thus far, and what can be done to help you reach your goals, remember to consider your spirit as much as you are considering your ovaries, uterus, endocrine and immune systems. Strive to maintain a well-functioning HPO Axis. Open the communication between your Heart and your Kidneys. Check in and connect to your own Heart.

Stress and Emotions:
This is truly where TCM shines! The relaxation and improvement in overall well-being reported in clients undergoing regular acupuncture treatments is extraordinary. From a strictly traditional Chinese medical

perspective, it is essential to determine the precise characteristics of the presenting 'stress', since each requires a unique treatment. Therefore it is important to define your stress. It has become a 'catch all' term for any physical or mental-emotional extreme (i.e., marathons, surgery, work pressure, anxiety, depression, etc.) and this raises a point which I need to be absolutely clear about: the stress associated with infertility may be one of the most profound emotional strains a woman will ever experience, and it will manifest in various ways for different women. Talking to someone during this trying time to identify specific areas of stress and its manifestations is a healthy way to strategize solutions.

- <u>Pressure points</u> - Learn and use pressure points known to relieve stress and anxiety. This is effective and easy. (see Step Eight)
- <u>Sleep</u> - When times are tough, take control of the few things you actually have control over. Get enough quality sleep so your body can best handle the assault that results from excess stress.
- <u>Nurture healthy friendships</u> -This is particularly important for women. If you have withdrawn from your girlfriends then it is time to put a little social time back into your calendar. Whether they offer a compassionate ear or just a fun distraction, they are definitely worthwhile.
- <u>Breathing</u> - Tie a string around your finger, seriously. I wear a ring every day of my life that is meant to do nothing else but remind me to breathe. Make it a reminder to slow down and take a deep breath. Incorporate deep breathing into an aspect of your life that you do regularly so that it becomes programmed at an instinctual level with practice. This will change the course of your health for the rest of your life. I deep breathe together with every client with every acupuncture needle I insert. This induces relaxation and creates a connection to potentiate its healing effects. This

ensures I take many deep breaths with every week that passes. Find something that works for you (i.e., each time you wash your hands or open a door) and install this ritual.

- Exercise - The stress-relieving chemicals released through exercise are unparalleled. When we are most stressed is usually when we feel paralyzed, but the opposite is what is needed to feel relaxed, happy and whole again.

Assisted Reproductive Technology (ART) Support:
When a woman decides to embark upon Assisted Reproductive Technologies such as In Vitro Fertilization (IVF), it can be assumed that the fertility journey has already been substantial. When I support a woman or couple preparing for or going through IVF, a heavy focus is placed on the improvement of patient experience by regulating emotions and reducing stress. Acupuncture is used extensively for the promotion of blood circulation through the reproductive organs to improve ovarian and uterine response to IVF medications. This is also a primary focus of treatment. It is important to choose complementary treatment options that are sustainable for you and choices you can realistically implement for the weeks or months leading up to retrieval and embryo transfer (see Step Eight). The following are a few simple choices we recommend:

- Guided relaxation/meditation - These can be fertility specific or just stress relieving. Anji online, Circle + Bloom, Dan Gibson, Jon Kabat-Zinn, and Deepak Chopra are just a few you could try.
- Castor oil packs, femoral massage, & foot soaks - Create a new nightly routine. These three practices encourage blood flow to your reproductive organs.
- Pressure points for stress relief - Applying pressure or massage to specific points on the body

can help combat the effects of stress.

- Sleep - The importance of sleep cannot be overstated. This is when the body gets a chance to regenerate and nourish itself. Make getting enough quality sleep a priority.
- Reducing workload - When we are not 25 but want our body to act this way, we must give ourselves the time required to nurture oneself, to slow down and conserve vital energy and focus for reproduction.
- Acupuncture - A burgeoning body of evidence displays the benefits of using acupuncture in conjunction with IVF cycles, both in the weeks prior and on embryo transfer day (see Step Nine for references).

Obesity:

If you are overweight, above all else, this is the area that should be tended to. The time is now to make the commitment to the lasting change required to lose weight. Often losing just a few pounds, or dropping your BMI (Body Mass Index) just a couple points is enough to get you to your goal. Do all the research you can and find all the help you need to make this happen. It is well known and accepted that being overweight or obese drastically reduces your chances of falling pregnant and carrying a healthy pregnancy to term. Quite possibly the most important element behind your success is having the proper support around you; do not underestimate the powers of your peer group*. Please refer to the exercise below and make the changes necessary with the company that you keep. Start today.

TCM can help reduce insulin resistance, regulate appetite, and encourage lipolysis (the breakdown of fat) which will help the body to lose weight and result in improved ovarian function and egg quality, translating into greater success rates both naturally and with IVF.

Since your weight management is largely in your control, you CAN do it, and it is simply choices and willpower that are needed to surmount the daunting task of weight loss. Perseverance, commitment and proper medical management is absolutely required.

- <u>Diet</u> - So important we gave it its own chapter.
- <u>Move</u> - It's that simple. Sometimes it might be better to not call it exercise. Physical activity is key, raising your heart rate, sweating, and possibly most important enjoying yourself. Aerobic target heart range is optimal for fat burning.
- <u>Willpower</u> - The ingredient of the recipe that holds the rest together. Coaching, public accountability and Chinese herbal medicine are all fantastic tools to utilize when needing to cultivate willpower.
- <u>Portions</u> - There may be many reasons for the obesity epidemic, but the only action that breeds obesity is the overeating of empty calorie foods. First of all, if necessary, reduce meal portion sizes.
- <u>Why</u> - The element which trumps willpower, is the reason. If your 'why' is strong enough, you'll find any way possible to achieve your goal. Keep yourself focused on losing weight and its correlation with having a family.

An Exercise:

Support System*: One of the most important things you can do to ensure your accomplish your goals and fulfill your dreams is to develop a support system. It is well accepted that we become very much like the five people we spend the most time with. Take a second to list these people here:

1. _____
2. _____
3. _____
4. _____
5. _____

Now ask yourself, are these people providing the support and inspiration you need to ensure you are constantly motivated to be moving toward your goals, to avoid self-sabotaging choices, to grow into the new you and write your new story? If the answer is no, then what I have to say is simple; choose different people to spend your time with. This could be key to unlocking your true fertility potential.

Thyroid Conditions:
The reason it is so important that the thyroid is healthy before conception is that the demands on the gland increase with pregnancy. The thyroid gland regulates metabolism and if it is already deficient then this increased strain may result in inadequate vital functions associated with the thyroid, often ending in miscarriage. The liver is required for the conversion of thyroid hormone and estrogen into a form that the body can use and eliminate. If the liver function is poor then proliferative estrogen is allowed to accumulate in the body lending itself to the growth of ovarian cysts, fibroids, endometriosis and reproductive cancers. Reproductive-related conditions that seem to increase the incidence of thyroid issues include: insulin resistance, PCOS and estrogen spikes caused by environment, medication or birth control pills.

- Liver cleanse: *A large percentage of thyroid hormone conversion into a usable form by the body is done by the liver. Liver health is also imperative for the proper conversion of many other hormones important to reproductive health. See the diet section on recommendations for liver health and avoid alcohol and other stressors on your liver.*

- Gut flora: *Sufficient gut flora, or the friendly bacteria found in probiotics, is necessary to convert thyroid hormones so they are usable by the body. I recommend taking non-dairy probiotics that are in an acid resistant capsule. Do not sacrifice quality when it comes to probiotic supplements.*
- Thyroid Peroxidase antibodies (TPO): *90% of hypothyroid cases in North America are estimated to be due to Hashimoto's, an autoimmune disorder involving the destruction of the thyroid. Keep your immune system and overall health in shape by taking your Vitamin D, probiotics and fish oils. Ask your doctor to run Anti-TPO blood work to see if you have an autoimmune thyroid issue.*
- Gluten & casein: *The protein in gluten that the immune system attacks when people are sensitive to gluten is chemically similar to TPO. So when gluten sensitive or celiac women eat wheat or other gluten containing grains, the activation of the immune systems attack on both the gluten protein and TPO is increased. It is also said that casein, a protein in dairy, also may cause the same issue. Therefore, women with Hashimoto's disease should eliminate dairy and gluten completely from their diet.*
- Iodine supplementation: *Use caution with iodine supplements as they could increase inflammatory damage done to the thyroid if the hypothyroid condition is actually Hashimoto's autoimmune thyroiditis. Iodine increases the production of the TPO enzyme that stimulates thyroid function, which under normal hypothyroid conditions is beneficial, but since the immune system is actually*

attacking the TPO enzymes in Hashimoto's,
increasing the amount of TPO by supplementing
with iodine could increase the immune response
and cause even more inflammation and destruction
to the thyroid tissue via immune attack.

Setting attainable goals will keep you on track and restore a sense of control. During a time that can feel like so much is out of your hands, achieving the smallest of goals is often a much needed boost of empowerment. Small, simple commitments over time create the changes we desire in life.

"Be kinder than necessary, for everyone you meet is
fighting some kind of battle."
~T.H. Thompson and John Watson

Story
Sally P.

"After two years of trying unsuccessfully to have a baby, I knew something was wrong. My periods had always been very irregular and I was frustrated because my family doctor would not refer me to a fertility specialist until we'd been trying for at least two years.
Finally, we were referred to the Pacific Centre for

Reproductive Medicine (PCRM) and started on Clomid. After four cycles without success, I wanted to get more aggressive with our treatments since we are not getting any younger. I came across a Yinstill brochure in the waiting room at PCRM and made an appointment. I had seen two acupuncturists before meeting the Yinstill team. One, for my migraines was helpful, but the second who focused on fertility, made me feel awful about not being able to conceive. When I would tell her how much she was hurting me, she would actually tell me that if I wanted a baby, I had to suffer. I felt discouraged and guilty. I felt like it was my fault we couldn't have a baby because I couldn't handle the suffering and pain. I thought there was something wrong with me-- that I was the problem. I was severely depressed at the time and had to take a leave of absence from work.

In spite of my bad experience with my previous acupuncturist, I was willing to try again with someone new. Luckily, Dr. Pentland was encouraging, extremely understanding and supportive. I felt like he really cared about me instead of seeing me as just another patient. I always enjoyed going into the clinic; it was a time for me to relax rather than feeling like I was going in for medical treatments. Spence made me feel confident and hopeful again and my husband and I truly believe that the treatments I received from Yinstill helped us on our journey to parenthood. I am forever grateful to Spence and Harris for not only the treatments but also their kindness and support throughout.

When I met Spence, we had just started our first IVF and I was feeling hopeful for the first time. Our treatment plan was to help my body work harmoniously with all the fertility drugs. The first round of IVF was not a success and I saw Spence sporadically after that but then I decided to get serious and do everything I could to make it work. I started going regularly once a week and also had a transfer day session with Spence. Sadly, that cycle didn't work either. By our third and final IVF though, I was going religiously twice a week and had a transfer day session. I was also more conscious of what I was eating. I ate healthier and more regularly and took some more time off work so I could be as relaxed as possible for the big day. It worked and I became pregnant!

Throughout our whole journey, seeing friends get pregnant and have kids was definitely painful. I felt like I was letting my husband down. I hated my body for not cooperating and doing what a woman is supposed to be

70

able to do naturally. It was a lonely journey because at that point, we were still very private about our struggles and there was no other couple we knew of that were going through the same thing. I felt that life was very unfair to us, we are good people and we did not deserve this. The pain of seeing friends get pregnant and have children did not disappear until we got pregnant ourselves. There were good and bad days but overall, I think our struggles with fertility have brought my husband and I closer together. If we can survive this, we can survive anything, even raising a child!

My treatment at the clinic with Spence and Harris made me more hopeful and less negative. I knew that we were doing everything we could to make it work and if it didn't, we had tried our best and that's all we can ever do.

Our son was born in July 2013. Even after I was pregnant, I continued to see Spence and Harris for my morning sickness. I would receive emails from both of them from time to time to check in and see how we were doing. I am a huge proponent of TCM and would recommend anyone trying to conceive to go see Spence. There are no immediate plans for us to have more children but if we change our mind, I would not hesitate to go back to Yinstill.

I can't describe what it is like to be a parent to our amazing miracle baby. I tear up thinking how much we've always loved him, before he even existed. It was a very difficult journey to get here but we would do it all over again to have him. Watching him learn new things every day is a gift and seeing him smile when he sees us is just incredible."

"Be thankful for what you have; you'll end up having more. If you concentrate on what you don't have, you will never have enough." ~Oprah Winfrey

Distraction

Learning this simple principle changed my life. It really made me become clear on exactly what it is I need to be doing with each and every moment of every day so that I ensure the accomplishment of my goals and dreams and live a happy fulfilled life. This simple principle is to avoid distraction. We are bombarded with distractions, from social media, email, television, shopping, and other peoples' agendas are just the tip of the iceberg. We live in a society where we pride ourselves on being busy. If you ask 10 people today how they are doing, I would guess that at least eight of them will mention how busy they are in their response. Five of those eight may admit that they are busy being distracted, actually doing very little to deeply fulfill themselves and live the life they want to live. This is not their fault, as most people have not been taught how to sit down and take the time to get crystal clear on the way they want to feel, the things they want, and to create a vision for their future.

Getting clear is the first step to success. Set precise detailed goals today. The second is prioritizing the skills, character, and tasks that are necessary to accomplish your goals. Then finally and most importantly, get rid of all the distractions in your life. This means everything that is not a part of your list of priorities has to be eliminated or delegated. This is a pearl of wisdom exampled by many successful people. I also want to emphasize that focusing your life in such a way sets you up to become an expert in whatever it is you prioritize, but it also means that you have to leave the notion that you can be great at many things behind. This notion is one of childhood dreams and is responsible for keeping people on the path to mediocrity.

You are extraordinary; let your light shine.

Do not underestimate the power of gratitude. It is a natural law that being grateful for what you have will attract more abundance. When you are grateful, it is impossible to be angry or scared; try it. Make sure you thank the divine each day for the baby that you will soon be blessed with.

"Give thanks for unknown blessings already on their way."
~Native American prayer

Chapter Task:

List your top three health related goals:

1. _____

2. _____

3. _____

Write down any questions you still have about goal setting:

_____

_____

_____

_____

_____

Now go and find answers to these questions!

Step Three

Self-Monitoring:

Learning to pay attention to your body's signals

"When we're willing to listen to our bodies and begin trusting ourselves as much as we trust outer authorities, all the rules change. And so does our biology. Statistics no longer apply to us. We enter the realm of miracles and undreamed-of possibilities." ~Dr. Christiane Northrup, author of Women's Bodies, Women's Wisdom

---

I had a favorite old Chinese teacher during my TCM studies that imparted simple but wise words to us. He said, "Your body is your best friend, listen to what it is telling you!" That is the premise of self-monitoring and fundamental to working together with your TCM doctor.

In this step, we will discuss what to look for and what it means.

At most clinics, like Yinstill, new patients are asked to fill out an intake questionnaire so it is helpful for you to have observed yourself thoroughly. As treatment continues, tracking changes as you get healthier will help treatment continue on an effective path.

No one has a better knowledge of your body and what is going on with it than you. If you pay attention, your body will tell you everything you ever wanted to know. *If* you pay attention.

Some things to watch:

Menstrual cycle

One of the most important things to understand as a woman, particularly when you are trying to conceive a child, is your monthly cycle. Ovulation can and should be carefully tracked in order to know exactly when the ideal timing to have intercourse is. But beyond that, your period and vaginal discharge can tell you a lot about what is going on with your body. By tracking the color, consistency, pain and PMS symptoms you will be able to give your doctor a full picture of your health. Rich, red blood indicates that it is well oxygenated and full of nutrients indicating a healthy environment for an egg to implant. Many women view their periods as an inconvenience or maybe even something they dread every month, yet they are truly a gift. They cleanse your body every month and give you valuable information about what is going on inside.

Ideally, a woman's cycle should be of moderate volume for 2-4 days then taper off for 1-3 days. Blood should be fresh looking in color with minimal brown and black or extreme brightness. It should be neither too thick or too watery in consistency and contain minimal clotting or tissue.

The most common complaints I see fall under the category of Qi and Blood blockage, which acupuncture is typically very effective for. After addressing the primary complaints I hear, including stress, tension and irritability, I address clotted menstrual blood. This is a symptom that is closely connected to fertility and as you can see in the statistics below, very common.

Top menstrual symptoms reported at Yinstill:

95% - clotted menstrual blood:

(38% small, 47% medium, 16% large)
78% - stress
74% - neck / shoulder tension
69% - PMS cramps
66% - PMS breast tenderness
64% - PMS bloating
61% - PMS moodiness
58% - irritability/impatience

Menarche (onset of menses)

According to TCM, and in my clinical experience, menarche starting at 14 years of age or older often seems to indicate a reproductive essence deficiency (Kidney Yin / Yang), especially if having difficulty conceiving. Conversely, the onset of menses too early in life (the age of 10 or earlier) shows possible involvement of environmental causes of hormone imbalance, and from a TCM perspective, excessive Heat. So ideally, a woman's cycle should commence around the age of 11-13.

Cycle length (based on an average of 28 days)

Typically, a woman's cycle should consistently fall between days 26-32 every month (that said, slightly longer cycles can be quite normal and fertile for many women). If your cycle varies from this, it is one of the first things to get on track for optimal fertility. Don't worry if you're not there yet though. A combination of diet (as detailed in Step Five), acupuncture and exercise will make a difference and maximize your chances of conception.

So that you can cross reference your symptoms with the Diet and TCM chapters, here is a brief summary of what your cycle may be telling you.

Always early (less than 26 day cycle)
This is caused by an overall deficiency of the body known as Qi deficiency, an accumulation of Heat (possible

inflammation), or poor blood circulation causing blockage known as Blood Stasis.

Always late (more than 32 day cycle)
May indicate a deficiency or blockage caused by ineffective digestion and poor production of blood (blood deficiency). This is often accompanied by poor circulation of blood and body fluids known as Blood Stasis and/or Dampness.

Irregular (a combination of early and late)
Irregular cycles are often a result of extreme emotions also known as Qi stagnation. It can also be caused by an overall imbalance of health or lifestyle which causes irregular nourishment to the reproductive organs, manifesting as a body with disorganized cycles. Multiple TCM patterns are often involved.

Blood

Volume
Most women observe this by the number of days they bleed and thus the type/amount of tampons or pads they use. The usual amount of blood loss per period is 10 to 35 ml. Each soaked normal-sized tampon or pad holds a teaspoon (5ml) of blood. That means it is normal to soak one to seven normal-sized pads or tampons ("sanitary products") in a whole period (http://cemcor.ubc.ca).

A heavy flow shows an overall deficiency of the body (Qi Deficiency), and/or accumulation of Heat (possible inflammation).

When periods are very light, it most often points toward ineffective digestion and poor production of blood (Blood Deficiency), and/or poor circulation of blood and body fluids causing blockage (Blood Stasis, Cold and/or Dampness).

78

Colour
In general, menstrual blood should not be purple, brown or black as these all denote poor circulation of blood and body fluids and cause blockage (Blood Stasis, Cold and/or Dampness). Very dark red or extremely bright red blood often points toward accumulation of Heat (possible inflammation). Diluted pink or pale blood most often implies poor production of blood (blood deficiency).

Consistency
Thick blood is due to accumulation of Heat (possible inflammation). Thin watery blood is due to an overall deficiency of the body (Qi Deficiency) and poor production of blood (Blood Deficiency). Clotted blood is most often due to emotional circumstances (Qi Stagnation) and/or poor circulation of blood and body fluids causing blockage (Blood Stasis, Cold and/or Dampness).

Pain

Ideally, a woman's cycle should not have any pain but most often there is slight cramping both before and during the first couple days of a woman's period. This is considered normal but pain before or during menses is almost always due to poor blood circulation causing blockage (Blood Stasis from various causes). Pain around ovulation denotes poor circulation of body fluids causing blockage (accumulation of Dampness).

PMS

As a rule, a woman's premenstrual phase should not bear symptoms that drastically affect her quality of life. From a TCM perspective, almost all premenstrual symptoms have their root in Qi stagnation, which often has emotional causes at its root. Being overly emotional, breast tenderness, bloating, nausea and headaches can all be regulated, at least to some degree by ensuring smooth flow of Qi in the body.

Cervical Fluid (vaginal discharge)

By paying attention to your discharge, you will have a much clearer understanding of when you are ovulating. The body gives clear signs that this event is most likely taking place, though the only true measure of ovulation is pregnancy.

Approximately 10-16 days before the onset of menstrual bleeding, a woman's cervix (the opening to her uterus) will open to allow sperm through. When this happens, it produces a translucent, slippery and stretchy fluid that is an ideal medium for sperm to swim in. It also changes the acidity or alkalinity (pH) of the vagina, and contains nutrition for the sperm in order to sustain them on their long journey toward the fallopian tube where they court the egg. Think of the cervix as being in charge for creating the mood for romance.

Checking your cervical fluid is easy; no need for any tools other than your fingers and eyes. You can start monitoring once your monthly bleeding has stopped. After you have observed your body for a couple of cycles, pre-ovulation fluid will be obvious. Here is what you are looking for:

1. A slippery consistency. This provides natural lubrication for intercourse. Some women report a wet sensation.
2. A transparent appearance that resembles raw egg-whites. This is due to higher water content which makes swimming easier for sperm.
3. The fluid should stretch when examined between the fingers and not appear tacky like lotion. The lotion-like cervical fluid is too dense for sperm to swim in.

For some women, examining discharge is very easy, since

there is plenty to observe on her underwear. For others, it may be necessary to insert a finger into the vagina to check if smaller amounts are present around the cervix.

Fertile pre-ovulation fluid is over 90% water and not only looks and feels like semen, but is its best friend on the long journey toward penetration of the egg. A few reasons for this include:

> *Lubrication.* Glycerol amounts increase during sexual excitement and around ovulation. This is thought to be responsible for the lubricating qualities that define these important reproductive events.

> *Vaginal pH.* Reducing the acidity of the vagina helps sperm survive, which is a natural occurrence around ovulation. High acidity kills sperm and other invaders, which is very beneficial, except when ovulating and trying to conceive. Pre-ovulatory cervical fluid lowers vaginal pH. If this does not happen naturally; lubricants like Pre-seed will help.

> *Swimming.* It is easier to swim in water than lotion. The consistency of this fluid is much more conducive to motility.

> *Food.* Sperm needs to eat. Components in the pre-ovulatory cervical fluid such as calcium, sodium, potassium, glucose, amino acids, zinc, copper, iron, manganese, & selenium, give the sperm what it needs to thrive.

Healthy pre-ovulatory cervical fluid is a very important part of the fertility equation. The interaction of sperm and cervical fluid must be harmonious for success with conception. In many cases, women are not producing adequate amounts if any, but fortunately that can be remedied in the following ways:

1. Use Pre-Seed sperm friendly lubricant. Currently, it is the only lubricant on the market proven to mimic the composition and functions of a woman's natural fertile cervical fluid.
2. Drink lots of water with lemon and/or coconut water.
3. Use Traditional Chinese Medicine and acupuncture to help restore balance to body fluid levels.

LH Ovulation Strips for Tracking Fertility

The LH Ovulation Strip is a urine test that is fast and easy. It is used to predict when you are having your luteinizing hormone (LH) surge. Since it is one of the most reliable predictors of ovulation, it is my recommended method when determining the fertile window of the menstrual cycle. Some new ovulation urine strips are also measuring estrogen hormone levels, which is not necessary for the purpose of trying to conceive.

These strips are perfect for timing intercourse as they produce a positive result 12-36 hours before ovulation. They can also help verify a lack of ovulation.

It used to be that the most common way of monitoring your fertile days was to chart your basal body temperature. This involved taking your temperature every morning before getting out of bed and observing its fluctuations. A dip, then spike in temperature meant you had probably ovulated. Unfortunately, there were a few shortcomings with this method. First, there are other factors that can cause a temperature spike such as stress, fever, poor sleep, alcohol consumption etc. More importantly, the temperature spike usually occurs 12-24 hours *after* you ovulate, making it too late for intercourse by the time a temperature change is detected.
You are actually considered to be at peak fertility in the

two days preceding ovulation, which is why you may have noticed your body producing the fertile cervical mucus before this. Sperm can survive inside your body for about 3-5 days, so having intercourse in these two days before egg release can make for the best chances of having sperm and egg meet. After being released, an egg lives for about 6-24 hours, after which it will dissolve if it isn't fertilized. So if you are getting your important indicator 6-24 hours after the fact, as with basal temperature monitoring, you've missed the window.

When your egg is mature and it produces a sufficient rise in estrogen levels, your pituitary gland is triggered to release a surge of luteinizing hormone (LH). This tells your body it's ready to ovulate. The increased LH (as measured on the LH ovulation urine test strips) triggers the release of the egg, which occurs about 12-36 hours after the surge. Since nothing other than impending ovulation triggers an LH surge, this method provides a clear message that your most fertile days have arrived.

Although using the LH ovulation strip is a great way of finding out when your best chance of conception may be, having regular sex (i.e., a few times per week or every other day) mid-cycle maximizes your chances of conception.

NOTE: *When purchasing these tests, please look further than your local drugstore as the price of ovulation test strips is unbelievably high. There are less expensive sources (for example, at Yinstill, we buy them in bulk so we can sell for a reduced rate).*

Bowel Movements

As embarrassing as this is for some people to talk about, it is one of the central indicators to a deeper understanding of what is happening for you internally. Your bowels are an expression of health, mainly digestive, but also may be great indicators of other underlying problems that should be investigated. What comes out dictates pretty clearly what's going on inside. So before you flush, take a peek!

The Bristol Stool Scale is a system created to standardize the appearance of stool so that reporting to your physician is easier.

Book Suggestion

If you want to learn more about the ways your body displays its reproductive health, have a look at Taking Charge of Your Fertility by Toni Weschler. It goes into great depth regarding basal body temperature charting and cervical positioning.

So, what is normal? According to TCM:

- 1-2 bowel movements per day is average.
- Without extreme urgency or incontinence.
- Formed, not loose or dry bitty rabbit pellet stool.
- Easy to pass (no grunting!).
- No burning sensation.
- No pain.
- Not too foul smelling.
- No undigested food should be seen.
- No 'unfinished feeling' post movement.
- If they float they are fabulous and filled with fibre.
- Colored like a fawn (depending on what you've eaten).
- No sense of fatigue post movement.
- Should not see any oily residue floating on water in toilet.

If there is blood, it should be monitored to determine what the source is; fresh blood on toilet paper or in the toilet water around an otherwise normal looking stool is most often not cause for alarm, however blood from further back in the digestive tract will produce dark tarry stool, which could be as simple as an ulcer or something more serious. In any case, if there is blood, please consult your physician.

Sleep Patterns

There are a few areas that I have strong opinions on and this is one of them. Sleep is when your body nourishes itself. During deep rest is when the body has a chance to pay attention to the systems that might not take priority in a busy day. The reproductive system gets a shot at optimal nutrition and oxygen delivery that might be redirected elsewhere during stressful waking hours so make it a priority to get enough sleep.

Digestion

Since your body knows best, how you feel after a meal will tell you a lot about which foods are good for you, and foods which you might be sensitive or allergic to. Fatigue, gassiness and bloating may be some signs that your food choices aren't working for you whereas energy and vitality are signs that you should keep up the good work. Digestive issues can also be an indicator of stress so if you feel like you've been eating well but your digestion is still not optimal, you may want to consider slowing down and looking at the big picture. If you are not getting extraordinary nutrition from food, how can you expect your body to flourish?

Moods

Moods can be just that sometimes but, more often than not, if you take a minute to assess what got you into the mood you're in, it can be a good indicator as to what's going on around you that may need your attention.

Conversely, a positive mood can let you know that the company you're keeping, your exercise routine or the way you spent your day is nourishing you.

Basal Body Temperature (BBT)

If your cycle is irregular, tracking basal body temperature (BBT) will allow for a better idea of what is going on internally but it is not my favorite way to predict ovulation since temperature range varies for individuals and can indicate not just fertility but thyroid or progesterone deficiencies, coldness or heat. The stress caused by taking ones temperature first thing every morning may outweigh the benefits of the information obtained. You be the judge. If waking every day and turning away from your partner to take your temperature is something you want to do then that is great; we can utilize this information. But if not, then please, unless your practitioner specifically believes that it is necessary, put the thermometer away. Although it is not necessary, many Doctors of TCM use the BBT chart to diagnose whether there is Heat in the follicular phase (day 1 to ovulation), if the body needs help ovulating and whether there are deficiencies in the luteal phase (ovulation to menstruation) that require supplementing. In my practice, I rely more on other feedback that the body gives us to determine direction of treatment and when the woman is ovulating.

If done properly and for an extended period, BBT charting is another indication of ovulation but since the small and not always apparent temperature dip and rise that happens is after your egg is released, it is too late to start trying once you see it. In conjunction with the rise in temperature, your 'fertile' cervical fluid will dry up and your cervix will close as the hope for implantation begins.

Libido

Sex drive can be an indication of everything from

ovulation to trouble within one's relationship. Oftentimes the stress of trying to conceive a child will affect your desire to be intimate with your partner and can be rectified by expressing this. Counselling can sometimes be the way to go or it may be as simple as taking the time to enjoy each other's company without focusing on reproduction.

There are 3-5 days of a woman's cycle where her libido rises and the cervix softens and retracts higher into the vagina, making sex much more comfortable by accommodating an erect penis.

Food Cravings

What you want and what you need may not align. It is not uncommon in the western world for us to eat when we are overworked or bored and especially when we are emotional. Some people refer to this as 'eating your feelings'. There are theories that suggest we might crave one thing when what we need is something entirely different, so do your best to be mindful of what you *really* want before consuming empty calories. Maybe a hug instead of a chocolate bar? And if that's not available, would a piece of fruit satisfy your desire for a donut? I never recommend deprivation though, so if you're sure you want a piece of cake, then have the cake. Just make sure you enjoy every morsel!

Skin

The largest organ on your body is a great indication of your health so observe it and learn what's up. How does it look and feel? If it's dry, drinking more fluids and eating more juicy fruits and veggies may help. Breaking out? Your body may be telling you it doesn't like what you've been eating or if you've improved your diet recently, it may be releasing old toxins. If your skin is oily, it may be an indication of Dampness or a sign that you're not assimilating nutrients. Yellow or grey? Get some fresh air! Your skin hides nothing so have a look and learn.

Trust your body. Your intuition in combination with your physical symptoms will guide you. And if you're having doubts or questions, that's what your TCM doctor is there for. This is a team effort.

...a little discussion regarding medical testing and self-monitoring

The 10 steps outlined in this book can be used alongside or completely independent of western biomedical care. That said, it is important to understand when it is time to ask your doctor to begin to run basic testing to rule out the obvious, like ensuring the fallopian tubes are clear via HSG (hystero - uterus, salpingo - tubes, gram - image), and whether there is any sperm being ejaculated during orgasm. Once these two tests are done, at least you can take a breath and move forward knowing that sperm is present and that it can get to the egg. When committed for enough time, you can make many changes in your life, overall health and fertility potential. However, blocked tubes and no semen are two conditions that will require western medical intervention.

After these basic tests are done, the second step is to help determine overall fertility potential. This involves the testing of FSH or follicle stimulating hormone (& estrogen), AMH or antimullerian hormone, and an AFC or antral follicle count. In my opinion, when these are done together, it gives us the most accurate picture of where a woman stands in her reproductive lifespan.

- *FSH (& Estrogen) - This is the hormone that is sent from the brain early in the menstrual cycle to tell the ovary to grow an egg. When blood tests show that this is elevated (i.e. > 10) then it can be concluded that the ovaries are not responding to this hormonal messaging very well, or the message is somehow not reaching the ovary. Estrogen must be tested in conjunction with FSH as high estrogen levels can artificially suppress FSH making it seem acceptable when it may not actually be the case.*

- *AFC - The antral follicle count is an ultrasound that images the ovaries and counts the follicles (fluid filled sacs in the ovaries which contain the eggs). A count of over 10 is great; 5 and above shows a moderate remaining fertility potential, and a count below 5 tells us that there is diminished ovarian reserve.*

- *AMH - A hormone produced by the ovaries that contributes to the deeper understanding of fertility potential that remains. Some health conditions reportedly can alter AMH results so this should never be used as a stand-alone test.*

Two studies regarding AMH (anti-mullerian hormone) are worth mentioning. A recent study published in the Journal of Endocrinology and Metabolism showed a 18% decrease in AMH levels in winter, which directly correlated to serum Vitamin D levels, and supplementing with Vitamin D prevented this seasonal change (Dennis, 2012). The other AMH study was published in Human Reproduction Oxford Journals and it showed significant changes in AMH levels throughout the menstrual cycle, AMH being at its highest concentrations mid follicular phase, between menses and ovulation (possibly something to consider when deciding when to give blood for your upcoming AMH test).

Story
Michelle K.

"Our fertility journey is a long and difficult one. We

started trying naturally in early 2007 when I was 31 years old and my husband was 35. After trying for more than a year, I went to see my family doctor to discuss it with her hoping she would refer me to a specialist, but she told me that nothing could be done as I was not considered infertile until trying for two years. I was really disappointed with her response as I had heard others say that after one year of trying, it is considered to be a problem. At that time, I felt that I was still young and thought that we were not in a great rush to have children so I didn't really research it and continued to try naturally. Two years passed and I had switched doctors, so I went to see him. I told him we had been trying for two years without success. He confirmed that I could have been referred to a specialist after one year. He referred me to my first fertility clinic but our first appointment wasn't until six months later. So we waited.

My blood work was normal (i.e., FSH, TSH, etc.) and I had excellent ovarian reserve. I was sent for a Laparoscopy diagnostic to see if there was anything inside that was a problem. I had to wait another six months for the Laparoscopy as it was covered under MSP. During the Laparoscopy, the doctor found and removed endometriosis so at that point that was considered to be the problem.

In the meantime, my husband was sent for sperm tests and the results showed his count was low. He was also sent for an ultrasound and the results showed that he had bilateral varicoceles. He was scheduled for embolization surgery to remove the varicoceles. The surgery was successful and his sperm quantity improved afterwards.

After we'd both recovered from surgery, we started IUI at end of 2010. We did a total of five IUI's but none of them were successful. All the pregnancy tests were negative. Our doctor was really surprised and thought that I would have gotten pregnant with the IUI's. She then determined that besides endometriosis and the male factor, there was also an unexplained reason for our infertility.

We decided to try IVF/ICSI in the summer of 2011. This time I had high hopes that I would be pregnant after my first IVF. I responded very well to the medications and had 15 follicles with 9 eggs.

The next day while I was waiting for the embryologist to call me to tell me how many eggs had been fertilized, the phone rang and it was my doctor instead. I knew it was not good news. She told me none of my eggs had been fertilized. I was very shocked and disappointed and so was she. She said this was the first time she had seen this.

The embryologist said that the reason for this was because the sperm lacked a mechanism to activate the egg for fertilization and suggested to add Calcium Ionophore to help with the fertilization. She said that there were some studies that used Calcium Ionophore when there was no fertilization with ICSI and results showed that it did help.

We attempted our second IVF in October, and this time I was really stressed, hoping the Calcium Ionophore would help. This time Dr. increased my medication but I didn't respond as well as last time and had to further increase my medication during injection. This time I only had nine follicles and three eggs. The Calcium Ionophore did help; one egg fertilized and was transferred on day three, however, the pregnancy test was negative.

Our third IVF/ICSI was done in the summer of 2012 at another clinic because our previous clinic's lab was going to be renovated (the clinic closed down in the end) and my doctor told me not to wait. I did have some concerns because I was worried that if this clinic doesn't use Calcium Ionophore then we will have no fertilization again. I voiced my concerns to the new doctor and he said that although he knows Calcium Ionophore helps, there is not much information on it. He suggested I try a cycle of IVF/ICSI and if there was no fertilization, he would offer me a second cycle for free and I would only be responsible for the medication at cost. We both agreed and off we went. I responded really well to medication and had seventeen eggs retrieved, fifteen were mature and five fertilized. I was really surprised and happy with the results. I didn't expect to have so many mature eggs and with five fertilized eggs, it gave me a thirty-three percent of the mature eggs being fertilized. The doctor said it was my best cycle, but for them five fertilized eggs out of fifteen, it was not great. He expected more for someone my age.

I ended up transferring two embryos on day five, reaching the blastocyst stage and even had one to freeze. Unfortunately the pregnancy test was again negative. We did the frozen transfer at the end of 2012 and that was negative as well.

After the failed frozen cycle, I wanted to start a fresh cycle of IVF/ICSI as soon as possible so I did my fourth cycle of IVF/ICSI right after the frozen cycle. For this cycle, we decided to try something new and added acupuncture to our transfer day. Studies showed that acupuncture immediately before and after transfer will increase chances of implantation so we had Dr. Pentland help us with the acupuncture. He was very nice and he had answered all the questions I had so I knew what to expect on that day.

That cycle, I didn't respond very well to medication so I had to increase it. I had a total of seven eggs retrieved with five mature and three fertilized. Although I didn't have as many eggs as last time, there was improvement in the fertilization, sixty-six percent of the mature eggs fertilized this time. I ended up transferring two embryos on day 3. This time they did not make it to day 5 blastocyst stage and I had none to freeze. The pregnancy test was negative as well.

After the failed fourth cycle in February 2013, I was waiting to be emotionally ready to start another cycle. However time was going by; it was the end of the year already and I still felt that I was not ready for another cycle. I was thinking to myself I couldn't continue to sit and do nothing and I remembered after my last failed cycle, Dr. Pentland said that we can discuss how acupuncture and Traditional Chinese medicine could help with my fertility journey, so I contacted him and went in to see him right before Christmas. My Traditional Chinese Medicine Pattern Diagnosis was: Qi & Phlegm stagnation with Spleen deficiency, Dampness accumulation and Heat. My husband was: LR stagnation causing Heat and King fire rising, Dampness accumulation below. Dr. Pentland suggested for us to come in for acupuncture once a week, take herbal medicine and some supplements. He also suggested for us to exercise regularly (now I try to do 30 minutes of exercise 3-5 times a week) and some diet recommendations (we have always eaten pretty healthy with all home cooked whole foods and lots of vegetables and fruit so we didn't need to make too many dietary changes). He recommended to try this for three to six months before considering going through another IVF cycle.

After a while, we did see some health improvements. I do look forward to our weekly acupuncture treatment as it is very relaxing. We are currently into four to five months of treatment right now and I have decided to start our fifth IVF/ICSI cycle next month. I feel that I am emotionally ready and I feel that after going through treatment with Dr. Pentland for a few months, I know our health is in an optimal state for the next IVF/ICSI plus I feel that I have tried my hardest this time. We went in to see our doctor again and this time he decided to change protocol. He told us because we had had four failed cycles and one failed frozen cycle that our chances this time would be even lower. He said we still need to have hope going into another cycle but to be realistic.

Every time we do an IVF/ICSI there are some improvements and it seems like we are closer to succeeding. I hope that this time we are successful and that my dream of becoming a mother will finally come true."

Chapter Task:

List three ways you will start monitoring yourself now:

1. _____

2. _____

3. _____

Write down any questions you still have about self-monitoring:

_____

_____

_____

Now go and find answers to these questions!

<u>Step Four</u>

Nurturing Your Spirit

Looking inside to get the whole picture

"What's meant to be will always find a way." ~Trisha Yearwood

---

S pirit can be a tricky thing to define and as such it can often be the last thing that people address when having reproductive challenges. I suggest you make it a top priority, however, as it is not only linked to physical health but quite often the cause of it. For me, spirituality comes in many forms, but I can boil it down to a nurturing of two values: growth and contribution.

Are you contributing in some way, making the world a better place? Are you growing as a person with new skills, learning from your mistakes, or looking past self and following the wisdom of something divine? It is also very important that you take the time to look at how you are feeling on a deep level, the nuts and bolts. How happy are you in your life as a whole? Do you feel like you have a purpose and if so, are you fulfilling it? Do you like your job or are you staying there because the benefits are attractive for when you get pregnant? Is the desire to have a baby putting a strain on your relationship?

Go back to church or temple regularly. Find time to meditate. Spend more time in nature. Volunteer for a worthy cause. Find things that nurture your spirit and decide right now that you are going to (re)incorporate them into your life. The fulfillment you will be gifted with is beyond words, and something that could have profound effects on your fertility and spirit of your unborn child.

The process of getting pregnant, or rather struggling to get pregnant according to plan, can be very stressful. Whatever caused the difficulty in conceiving originally is now compounded with the immense stress that accompanies infertility. Women instinctually understand that stress is not good for reproduction, so this results in more stress and a frustrating cycle emerges. Sadly, in this sense, infertility may become its own cause.

Taking the time to balance the big picture with staying in the moment is key to a contented inner life and being self 'full'.

Stress

"Doing nothing is better than being busy doing nothing."
--Lao Tzu

Stress is such an umbrella term these days. Since it covers everything from being overworked to emotional strain within a relationship or financial worries, all of us are bound to have some. It is how we deal with it that determines whether it becomes harmful.

There are mixed opinions as to whether stress has an effect on fertility but I question, how could it not? When someone experiences stress, the body releases a hormone called cortisol. Whether it's meeting a deadline, fighting with your spouse or being chased by a pack of hungry wolves, cortisol bubbles through our veins. In the past (like when you may have actually been being chased by wild animals), cortisol was essential for survival because it heightened the senses making us faster, stronger and keenly aware of our surroundings. When the imminent danger was gone, cortisol levels dropped and our body slowly went back to functioning regularly. In a modern day world, however, we sustain these levels for prolonged periods of time and *that* is where the problems start.

In situations of long term stress, health dangers are rampant. The body is not designed to sustain heightened cortisol levels and it causes trouble for the immune system. When there is trouble in the immune system, there is trouble everywhere. From colds to cancer to chronic fatigue, a weakened immune system plays a role. And what about fertility? How does a compromised immune system play a role there?

Think of your body as a very busy life. There is a LOT going on. You have to maintain a job, you've got your relationships, both personal and professional. There's your family, your social life, your health, maybe some travel, home maintenance and maybe that nagging little noise your car is making. You can't do everything at once.

You have to schedule your time wisely and prioritize. If work is hectic, your social life might suffer and if you have to fly home to look after your sister's kids while she's sick, your job is going to have to take a back burner for a couple of weeks.

Your body is the same. It has a lot to do and it has to decide what is most important. When stress is a long term thing, reproduction is not the priority. Instead of making sure your reproductive organs are getting enough circulation, blood flow is going to the heart because the cortisol is telling it that there is imminent danger and it needs to beat faster.

Your body is highly intelligent and its job is to keep you alive. Producing offspring is secondary to the number one job - looking after you. When YOU are healthy, then your body is free to think about creating someone else.

Some stress is inevitable. We are all susceptible to the traffic jams and holiday dinners and trips to the dentist. Dealing with stalled fertility can be a huge stress. How do you avoid letting those instances make your cortisol levels rise?

Figuring out your stressors is a good place to start. I suggest making a detailed list of everything in your life that makes you a little edgy. Include both significant and minute from running late for an appointment to fighting with your spouse. Then qualify this list into two additional categories--things you have control over and things you do not.

For the list of things that you have control over, set some goals for yourself to move on from those stressful situations. Could you reduce the frustration that traffic causes by using public transit? Is there someone that you need to have a heart-to-heart with to get through a strained relationship? Can you delegate some of your duties elsewhere to free up some time for yourself?

And for the list of things you don't have control over, I suggest you pair them with a third list. A list of everything that makes you feel relaxed and happy. It might be a deep breath to gain perspective and some dedication to reprogramming your reactions, but a hot bath, a run along the seawall or a cuddle with your dog are also guaranteed to combat stress. If it makes you feel good, it has the opposite effect that cortisol does. The chemicals released from pleasurable activities actually boost your immune system and like everything in Chinese medicine, good health is about finding balance.

How stress impacts fertility is not completely understood but high levels of stress can prevent pregnancy and affect a woman's chance of conceiving. What we do understand is that taking steps to manage stress provides a better quality of life during challenging times.

How stress impacts a fertility patient

For some, being unable to conceive breeds an obsession with pursuing anything and everything that might help, from prayer to vitamins to IVF. Others completely withdraw from life, loved ones and society as a whole. Either extreme must be addressed in order to accomplish their goal of creating a happy healthy family.

How to reduce stress

Proper stress management helps people feel more in control and can improve overall well-being.

In 2014, The American Society for Reproductive Medicine (ASRM) released a patient education fact sheet on stress and infertility. It talks about the unknown impact of stress on fertility, how stress impacts fertility patients, how to reduce stress, and how people can help loved ones or friends going through this difficult time.

Reducing stress can help bring a sense of clarity and aid women and couples in making better decisions for their health and fertility treatment options. It should be remembered that being stress free during fertility struggles is an unrealistic expectation, but finding ways to minimize stress and its detrimental effects is recommended.

Acupuncture, aerobic exercise, guided imagery, journaling, listening to music, massage therapy,

Stress and the Human Body

* In a prospective cohort study, a group of researchers from the U.S. decided to answer the question: Are women's stress levels prospectively associated with infertility? They measured bio markers (i.e., specific chemicals or hormones) for stress in their saliva and a perceived stress questionnaire in almost 400 couples. What they found was that when these bio markers and perceived stress were higher, the time to pregnancy was increased (Lynch, 2014).

* In a study done attempting to explain exactly how acupuncture helps with stress on a biological level, researchers found that it actually regulates the specific hormones associated with the biochemical reactions that take place in the body as a result of stress (Wang, 2014).

meditation, mind-body groups, mindfulness, progressive muscle relaxation, psychotherapy, self-help books, support groups, visualization, walking/hiking and yoga. These are just a few suggestions that could be a part of a stress management program.

How to help those who are struggling

Avoid telling them to 'just relax and you will get pregnant'. Compassionately asking how they are doing and listening is likely the most important thing you can do for your loved one. If you feel it timely and appropriate, gently offering valuable tools that may reduce stress, improve quality of life and bring back a regained sense of control may be very appreciated.

Meditation

"Muddy water, let stand becomes clear." ~Lao Tzu

Meditation is a practice that is becoming more and more prevalent in the western world even though cultures have been practicing it for ages. It is a very simple concept that can be extremely helpful for allowing an individual the opportunity to get in touch with their inner self. Here are the basics:

1. Sit comfortably in a warm, quiet place where you won't be disturbed.
2. Relax and pay attention to your breath. Take deep belly breaths that fill your abdomen.
3. Clear your head. When thoughts arise, gently let them go and bring your attention back to your breathing.

It may be a challenge at first but start small. Five or ten minutes a day will have an impact and you can increase the time you sit as you get more comfortable with your practice. Be patient with yourself. Thoughts will arise and that is normal. When you realize you are thinking rather than focusing on your breathing, just guide yourself back lovingly. Regular meditation will lower your blood cortisol levels and help ground your energy so that you can embrace the journey to parenthood calmly.

Take a Moment...or Two

Some people are intimidated by meditation; maybe it sounds too new-agey or you just feel you don't have time. If that's the case, I suggest a less rigorous form of mindfulness that can be done throughout your day and is much more simple.

Choose an activity that you partake in daily such as

washing your hands or having a glass of water or even opening a door. Each time that you do that activity, check in with yourself. Take a couple of deep breaths and consider for a moment where you're at emotionally, physically and intellectually. You don't have to address your feelings in any way nor judge them. Simply acknowledge where you are and what you're doing. Then, most importantly, smile and be grateful for all the wonderful blessings you have in your life. Be in the moment for that moment and then carry on with your day. Think of it as checking in with yourself the same way you would your partner or someone else you care about.

When mindfulness practices are done consistently, they become programmed to be a part of your instinctual makeup. Over time, they play a massive role in changing your life. It is the little things that make big differences.

Self-Care

"Sleep is the best meditation." ~Dalai Lama

Nurturing yourself is always important. This is even more crucial when you are wanting to become a parent. While it may be hard to define, spirit is always something that seems to thrive when you take good care of yourself. Self-Care means something different for everyone so I encourage you to find what works for you. A few favorites include: warm baths, alone time, time with friends and loved ones, exercise and regular massage; we will talk more about it in Step Eight.

Giving Back

Another way to nourish your spirit and to take your mind off things is to lend a hand to those that need it. Sometimes the best way to get out of our heads is to do something selfless. And again, putting others first can be great preparation for parenting. Helping someone in need not only gives us a sense of purpose, but will often induce gratitude for our own circumstances thus pulling us out of the rut of self-pity and frustration.

The American writer and philosopher, Ralph Waldo Emerson, put it best when he said, *"It is one of the most beautiful compensations of life that no person can sincerely try to help another without helping themself."* This is such a great quote that it needed to be put into the book twice!

Top Tip for Stress Reduction: Sit Down, Breathe and Think of Nothing
by Dr. Harris Fisher

Picture yourself sitting cross-legged on the floor, breathing rhythmically and thinking of absolutely nothing. This is you reducing stress and assisting your body in reducing inflammation. In the January issue of Brain, Behavior, and Immunity [1], there is an article that outlines a study that was done comparing the stress-reducing effects of an eight-week mindfulness-based stress reduction program (MBSR) and an eight-week active control health enhancement program (HEP) that included walking, balance, agility, core strength, nutritional education and music therapy.

The results of the comparison were enlightening and unexpected by the researchers. It appears that mindfulness meditation practices are as effective at stress reduction as the health enhancement program listed above, but also showed that meditation practice may be better at recovering from stress situations and actually reduces the inflammatory response associated with stress. For people that are physically unable to implement health enhancement activities, mindfulness meditation is an excellent alternative. For everyone else, it should be a complement to a healthy lifestyle and both of these practices should be a part of our daily routine.

Mindfulness meditation does not require a gym membership or special equipment and does not have to take a long time. You can do it anywhere and at any time during your day. In all the treatments that I offer at Yinstill, I give people the option of combining a guided meditation to their acupuncture experience. The effects of the acupuncture session can be sustained for several days with daily mindfulness meditation practice.

Story
Sukhy B.

My fertility issue was amenorrhea (an absence of periods). The doctors didn't really know what caused this but a couple of theories are it's diet or stress-related. I personally believe stress is the biggest factor so a big part of my recovery was learning how to manage stress. One of my most valued ways is yoga and it changed my life, but I'll get to that.

Since my periods were months apart (I had maybe 3 or 4 in a year) and we were eager to start a family, getting medical intervention and assistance was a priority.

In spite of my irregular menstruation, the first time I got pregnant it happened naturally after only 4 months of trying. Unfortunately I miscarried a set of twins close to the end of the 1st trimester. After that I never got pregnant naturally again.

I started taking Clomid, steadily increasing the dosage as the lower doses were ineffective. After a couple of increases in doses by my GP with no results, I was referred to a Gynecologist. She continued with Clomid for a while and then did some physical examinations, including a hysterosalpingogram; the dye test which revealed a blockage in one of the tubes. An endocrinologist at UBC was later unable to find any blockage and concluded that the dye itself may have cleared the blockage when it was flushed through my tubes. He then performed a laparoscopy which showed no issues and told us everything was in working order.

By that time, we had already been trying for a baby for about 5 years. I was feeling very frustrated by how slowly it was moving and that because I was still considered young, that the doctors seemed to be in no hurry. I didn't feel the same though; I was married and we wanted to start a family immediately. In hindsight, I'm glad I didn't get pregnant in my early twenties though because I have grown up so much since then, and I parent very differently now than I would've done then. I firmly believe everything happens at the perfect time. We waited 20 long years for our miracle babies. During that time I did a lot of growing up, mentally and most importantly, spiritually. I am wiser, more patient, and learnt a lot about raising children through observation of others and through reading and educating myself.

Next I began Ovulation Induction treatments which are one step less than IVF. Drugs are used to stimulate the ovaries to produce multiple eggs and then once the follicles are the right size, you are given a shot of HCG hormone to trigger ovulation. You are then left to go home and have intercourse, as per the schedule. This treatment meant enduring daily injections for days at a time and increasingly feeling the uncomfortable sensations of swollen ovaries to the point that by the time I was ready to ovulate, I was unable to walk briskly because it was just too painful. My ovaries would start off responding very slowly to the drugs and then boom, numerous follicles would start growing fast and furiously, and the ovaries would enlarge accordingly. Toward the end of the first round, my doctor almost cancelled the final shot to trigger the ovaries to release the eggs because I had overstimulation of the ovaries but being advised of the risk, we still went ahead. I was told to take it very easy, under the threat of complete bed rest. Thankfully my body recovered on its own.

Regardless of the challenges of this route, we persevered and became pregnant after the very first round of treatment, but it was short lived. The pregnancy was found to be tubal but resolved on its own, without surgery, thankfully.

Over a span of a few years we continued numerous more cycles of ovulation induction; I believe 12 in total, but all to no avail. There were no more pregnancies.

We would take time off in between to re-group, re-energize and re-focus. Needless to say, the desire to have children but the inability to accomplish it is very taxing on your body, mind, spirit and relationship. We went through all the emotions every couple having difficulty getting pregnant goes through. The heartache, the depression, the disappointment, and of course the questions: Why me? Why us? What did we do wrong? What are we being punished for? And the inevitable questions and suggestions from well-meaning family and friends.

At that point, the doctor said our options were basically to try IVF or just give nature another chance, since I was only 28 years old. We decided to give IVF a try because by now, we both wanted a baby so badly, and it seemed to have better odds. So I underwent a whole other batch of tests and work-ups in preparation for IVF. It was a few months before we actually had the treatment. All went well, I produced numerous eggs, but it still didn't result in a pregnancy. We went for a post-treatment follow-up with our doctor and he told us that approximately 50% of the

*eggs tested had an abnormal number of chromosomes.
Needless to say, this totally freaked us out. We didn't
pursue any more conventional medical treatments for 10
years after that.*

*During those 10 years, we didn't completely give up on
having children though. We tried Chinese medicine,
acupuncture and naturopathy. I said prayers, practiced
gratitude and most importantly, kept faith. I prayed and
meditated regularly. There were times when I wondered
whether I would ever have children, but I also continually
saw signs that it would happen. Things like people giving
me suggestions on what therapy to try, or telling me
stories of how others persevered on their journeys. To me,
these pieces of information were communications from the
Universe telling me not to give up. I occasionally checked
in with myself and asked why I wanted to have children to
make sure my reasons were coming from me, and not from
other people's expectations for me. What I came up with
was that I have a lot of nurturing and caring energy inside
me and I wanted to give that to a child. One thing that
really resonated with me was hearing Dr Phil say, when
you are pursuing something that seems to be eluding you,
look at what feeling or emotion it is that you are trying to
achieve by having that desire fulfilled, and then find other
ways to attain that emotion. Since I longed to be able to
buy baby things for my own children, I started buying
baby food, formula, diapers and donating them to the food
bank regularly. It helped me to live as though my wish
was already fulfilled, a recommendation I got from
reading The Secret.*

*The thing with natural therapies was, even though they
didn't help me conceive, they were benefitting my body
rather than taxing it like the other methods had. I was
eating healthier, taking supplements and integrating
exercise into my days. I discovered Bikram's Hot Yoga. It
was one of the best things ever to come into my life and*

actually, the most helpful as far as trying to correct my menstrual issue was concerned. After practicing the yoga for a few months, at least 4 times a week, consistently, I noticed my periods become a little more frequent. I was astounded, because absolutely nothing in the conventional or natural medicine had managed to accomplish that. I can't say enough good about it. Not only did it make that miraculous improvement, but I lost weight, my body firmed up and became flexible and strong, I had beautiful soft skin, slept like a baby and woke up totally refreshed and energized. I was enjoying the yoga and its benefits so much that I actually stopped thinking about actively pursuing getting pregnant, although secretly I would still hope every month that my period wouldn't come.

Ten years went by with the encouragement of a new family member, everything aligned and we decided we would try again.

This time when I went to see the doctor for our first appointment, I brought up the results of the quality of my eggs after the last IVF cycle. He told me that the results were totally normal and that 50% abnormality was not out of range, something we'd never heard before. It really helped us relax and feel better about undergoing IVF again. Everything was being aligned just perfectly for us to embark on this journey again.

We underwent another IVF cycle in August of 2008. I was in the waiting room towards the end of the cycle when a flyer caught my attention. It was about using acupuncture to enhance IVF treatments. I was already familiar with acupuncture and the flyer intrigued me so we decided to give it a try.

I was only able to get in 2 treatments prior to retrieval and then double treatment on the day of but lo and behold, it worked and we were pregnant again.

Unfortunately it was short lived; it turned out to be an ectopic pregnancy in the tube, which was missed by the ultrasound tech and the on-call doctor at the women's hospital. After waiting 2 hours to see her, she didn't seem to have the knowledge or desire to investigate my issue thoroughly. I was in excruciating pain but was told that since it was after hours and all the ultrasound technicians were gone for the day, that an ultrasound would only be performed in a life or death situation. She also said that she was having a hard time feeling anything through my abdomen 'because of all the fat'. My abdomen was enlarged, and yes there was some fat there but there was also a lot of fluid released from the ovaries. At 5'6" and 150 lbs., I don't think I was so fat that a doctor would have a hard time examining me. Needless to say, bedside manner is crucial and something I came to really appreciate with Dr. Pentland.

So we went home, dejected. I continued to take Tylenol for the moments of extreme pain. Ultimately, my tube ruptured and I ended up undergoing emergency surgery and losing my tube, as well as a considerable amount of blood.

My mental and emotional savior during that time was what I had read and learnt from The Power of Now by Eckhardt Tolle. I was able to remember as I was being wheeled into the operating room the power of surrendering to the moment and accepting what is. As soon as I totally accepted what was in that moment, I felt immensely lighter and able to move on with the healing process.

After picking ourselves up off the floor for the umpteenth time, and lots of encouragement from family and friends, we decided we weren't going to give up hope just yet; we would try just one more IVF cycle. I managed to convince my husband that we should still incorporate Acupuncture into our treatment as I was absolutely convinced it had helped with our last cycle and would do so again. I started seeing Spence in January 2009 on a regular basis, adjusted my diet a little and went back to doing my yoga classes 3-4 times a week.

In August, we started our fresh IVF cycle (prior to that we had 2 FET cycles, one of them resulted in a 'clinical' pregnancy, the other no pregnancy). This time I produced 35 eggs but even better than that, the quality of the eggs were excellent, the best I'd ever had. And our results just kept getting better; 70% of the injected eggs fertilized and all of them continued to blastocyst stage (Day 5)! We had never had such excellent results before. The only thing I can attribute these results to is the acupuncture as that is the only thing that was different in this cycle.

I had 3 embryos replaced at the Day 5 stage. Much to our delight, my first pregnancy test revealed a good level of the pregnancy hormone and the second pregnancy test showed the numbers increasing perfectly. I was feeling hopeful, far less anxious than previously and without the pain, discomfort and discharge of before.

My doctor sent me to a new ultrasound technician but he couldn't find the pregnancy. He told us that my uterus was inverted, and that this was a totally normal occurrence, and at some point it would come into the correct position but that the position it was in currently meant the ultrasound waves couldn't see it completely. They also did a vaginal ultrasound and didn't see anything out of the ordinary, so that was a bit of a relief.

Again we went home and waited for a second ultrasound. So much waiting!

That one was worth the wait. It showed us what we had been wanting to see for almost 20 years! 2 little blobs and

2 tiny specks of hearts beating. We were thrilled, cautiously thrilled, but still thrilled. It was one of the best days of our lives!

The remainder of the pregnancy went well. I continued with the acupuncture for the first trimester. I believe that helped keep my babies healthy and strong and myself as well. They delivered at almost 33 weeks, a girl and a boy, weighing 3½ lbs. and 4 lbs.

Even though they were a few weeks premature, they were very healthy, did not need any oxygen and were off their IVs within the first week. I attribute these results to the acupuncture.

I couldn't have asked for better results. When spending thousands of dollars on fertility treatments, a little more for Spence's acupuncture was soooo worth it. Even if pregnancy is not the outcome of all your efforts, it will benefit you in so many other ways.

Our little miracles just turned 4 and fill our days with joy, amazement, laughter and love. That doesn't mean we don't have challenges, but by the grace of the Universe, those are just moments in our otherwise wonderful days.

I would like to say to all of you reading this, looking for hope and successful stories: I know what you're going through, just don't give up hope, it's all we really have. I truly believe something good comes out of everything, absolutely everything that happens in our lives (even the not so pleasant stuff), and if being a parent is the best and right thing for you in this lifetime, it will happen. Don't worry about the when, the Universe times everything perfectly.

It'll happen at the perfect time.

Chapter Task:

List three things you will start to do today that will nurture your spirit:

1. _____

2. _____

3. _____

Write down any questions you still have about nurturing your spirit:

_____

_____

_____

_____

Now go find the answers to these questions!

Step Five

Curing Yourself with Diet and Supplements:

Looking inside to get the whole picture

"Tell me what you eat and I'll tell you what you are!"
~Anthelme Brillat-Savarin, 1826

There is a world of information out there these days about what a healthy diet consists of and it seems to be changing all the time. The abyss of rhetoric about what is healthy and what is not can be overwhelming but the important thing is to find what's right for you. If you are having digestive issues and you're not sure what the culprit might be, I suggest what the Chinese call the Qing Dan diet, which translates to clear and bland. You start with clear bland foods such as vegetable broth and build in other foods being mindful of how you feel along the way. It is a great way to see how your body reacts to different foods so that you can feed yourself accordingly.

There are trendy health foods that come and go, countless books to read and advice from everyone and anyone on what works for them, but again, like everything else in Chinese Medicine, I'd encourage you to find what works for you. Having said that, here are some basics that are pretty universal.

Relax

There is a lot to be said for the idea of sitting down with

115

friends or family to share a meal. It is a chance to check in with yourself and your companions wherever you are at in your day and to take a break. So often, food becomes a necessity that is rushed through and maybe not even considered as anything more than another task on your to-do list. This is not healthy. Instead, do your best to enjoy and appreciate your meals by relaxing and chewing thoroughly. Be grateful for the delicious food you are taking in and conscious of the nourishment it is providing for your body.

The Rainbow Diet

To keep it simple, try color-coding what you put in your body. Eat lots of colorful food; leafy greens, bright yellow squash and crisp red peppers are the way to go! All too often plates are piled high with brown, grey and white food. In general, colorless food is low in essential nutrients, processed and high in sugar, which results in frequent hunger as your body yearns for the nutrition not being provided. If you give your body what it needs, its cravings will be for more of the same rather than processed empty calories that make you sluggish and promote further poor choices.

Weight

I have seen many cases of women that are either overweight and underweight have trouble conceiving. Don't judge your weight by what you see in magazines but rather by what feels healthy to you. A combination of healthy diet and an appropriate exercise routine is always a recipe for success.

With regard to unhealthy weight and all other physical ailments, the philosophy of Traditional Chinese Medicine is to treat the root of the problem rather than the symptoms. The cause of all disease will fall into one of the following categories: improper eating habits, overwork, lack of physical activity or too much of it, external evils (virus, bacteria, toxins, etc.), excesses of emotion, climate or trauma.

In order to address the root of one's weight issue, we need to identify its cause and address it. If emotions are the root cause, which often they are, counting calories will get you nowhere. Instead, try counseling, coaching or hypnosis to help manage. And if emotions are not the root cause, with time they often become a contributing factor, so having someone to talk to can be very useful. If your job is stressful or your relationship is an unhappy one, these things will be reflected in your physicality. As well, taking steps to improve them will have a positive impact.

In conjunction with addressing emotional issues, Traditional Chinese Medicine (TCM) emphasizes the importance of cultivating willpower to overcome conditions such as overeating and laziness. Acupuncture and Chinese herbal medicine supplements the systems necessary for being proactive in one's life and to make healthy choices for mind and body.

The Male Factor

Unfortunately, I still see a lot of the responsibility for making changes falling on the women that are trying to conceive, when in fact, men are half of the equation and need to watch their diet as well.

Sperm quality is impacted greatly by what men put in their bodies. I'll get more in depth with the importance of sperm parameters in Step Ten, but here are a couple of easy tips gentlemen should adhere to that is based on numerous studies, as well as my own personal observations.

Avoid processed meats and dairy

A March 2009 study in Fertility and Sterility showed that poor semen samples were directly related to the intake and presence of products that may contain xenoestrogens or certain sex steroids (mostly in the saturated fats found in processed meat and dairy). If you consume animal products, stick to hormone-free and organic.

Eat more organic fruits and vegetables, both raw and cooked

If there is any doubt about the importance of organics, please read on to Step Seven where I get into specifics about various toxic pesticides and what they do to our bodies. The higher the antioxidants consumed in the diet, the better the sperm numbers and morphology (shape). Healthy Diet = Healthy Sperm.

Supplements

While the majority of your nutrients should be in your food, when that's not possible, I recommend supplementing. Like everything you put in your body, you must be critical when choosing supplements as they can be manufactured with cheap synthetics instead of premium organic whole food. The quality of your supplements play a major role in their effectiveness and in helping to correct the imbalance they were intended for. What is right for you will be determined by your practitioner but here are some suggestions and what they can be good for:

- Dietary cleanse - An anti-inflammatory dietary cleanse that will help you understand sensitivities and optimize liver function and hormonal balance.

As far as dietary cleansing goes, you want to create a healthy body in preparation for pregnancy. Cleansing for fertility is a great way to support the body and benefits overall well-being, immune and hormonal regulation, optimal liver kidney and bowel function and reproductive organ health.

- CoQ10* (ubiquinone, ubiquinol) - A naturally occurring enzyme in each of our cells that helps the mitochondria produce ATP (Turunen, 2004), or cellular energy. Recent research from Toronto, Canada shows that CoQ10 may improve egg quality (Bentov, 2013) through the mechanism of mitochondrial ATP enhancement - the same way some Chinese herbal medicines are thought to increase fertility, as well as being a heavily researched antioxidant extremely beneficial for heart health. Antioxidants such as CoQ10 (commonly seen in skin care products) are thought to slow down or even reverse your biological/cellular age and can be of great benefit when trying to conceive. CoQ10 has also been shown to improve sperm motility. Researchers from Spain recently performed a 'meta-analysis' (a study of existing studies on the particular topic of CoQ10 and sperm) and found a global improvement in sperm parameters (Lafuente, 2013). CoQ10 should be in a capsule that contains an oil base and is to be taken with food for optimal absorption. The ubiquinol form of CoQ10 is thought to be better absorbed than the ubiquinone form, but many companies today are patenting forms that are said to have better absorption rates, despite the actual form used.

*Currently there is insufficient evidence of CoQ10's safety during early pregnancy; avoid using.

- Omega-3 Fish Oil (EPA and DHA) - Regulates inflammation, promotes circulation and delivers required fats for the proper production of sex hormones - to help normalize your cycle. Reduces inflammation in the pelvic area which is especially important for fertility. Omega-3 fatty acids may reduce sensitivity to prolactin (which can suppress ovulation), increase cervical mucus to help the sperm reach the egg and blood flow to the uterus to help with development of the uterine lining. Strong caution should be taken when choosing a brand of fish oil. I recommend Nordic Naturals or Nutri-Sea in my practice as their quality control standards are amongst the highest in the industry. Testing for heavy metals, rancidity and purity, as well as ethical fishing practices should all be standard. In general, I also recommend oils high in EPA (an omega-3 fatty acid) when trying to conceive, then switching to oils higher in DHA (an omega-3 fatty acid) when pregnant. I also encourage the consumption of walnuts, avocados, olive oil and other alpha-linolenic acid (ALA) containing vegetables and nuts as a source of omega-3s (in addition to fish oil). If a client is a vegetarian, I simply recommend Udo's Omega-3 blend.

- B6/folate/B12 (homocysteine) - It is thought that women with Polycystic Ovary Syndrome (PCOS) or recurrent loss may have high homocysteine levels (a substance in our body that can cause problems with our circulatory system) due to conversion in the liver. B6, folate, & B12 in combination help convert homocysteine into a non-toxic substance and may help reduce the chances of miscarriage. Interesting to note, Metformin, a blood sugar regulating medication given to women with PCOS and insulin resistance, may actually increase homocysteine levels. This blend of B vitamins is safe and encouraged to be taken during pregnancy if you have tested positive for raised homocysteine levels, have experienced recurrent pregnancy loss or have been diagnosed with PCOS. Folate and B12 are also well known vitamins required for the production of blood and important in women who may suffer from Anemia, another possible cause of difficulty getting and staying pregnant

- Calcium D-glucarate, Indole 3 Carbinol - Both of these supplements have been researched for their use in the treatment of cancer as they aid the liver in the elimination of excess estrogens manufactured from excess adipose tissues or environmental toxins (which in some cases can encourage the growth of cancer). This mechanism may also be helpful in many reproductive health issues that have hormonal imbalance involving excess circulating estrogens (cysts, endometriosis, PCOS, fibroids, post administration of gonadotropic hormone medications used in fertility treatments such as IVF). This can also prevent cellular damage and benefits the body's immune system.

- Inositol (Vitamin B8) - Myoinositol has been shown to restore regular ovulation, lower insulin and decrease androgens. Also, can aid in the treatment of anxiety/panic attacks, insomnia, depression, mood regulation and high cholesterol. This is an important supplement for women with PCOS.

- N-Acetyl Cysteine (NAC) - Increase insulin sensitivity and lower androgen levels. A recent study using NAC on women with Endometriosis

(500mg 3x/day for 3 consecutive days per week, i.e., Monday to Wednesday, then a break for the remaining 4 days) showed reduced inflammatory and pain signaling factors, helped keep cells from becoming invasive, kept cysts from growing and even reduced their size (Porpora, 2013). NAC may also protect against health problems such as diabetes, reinforcing its use in PCOS women.

- Vitamin D - For general overall health and immune function. Vitamin D works synergistically with other vitamins and minerals (without Vitamin D, calcium won't be absorbed in the hard tissues like the bones and teeth which is essential if you want to get pregnant). It also supports the 'killer cells' of the immune system which may lower your risk of cancer cell growth and help regulate autoimmune conditions. Additionally, Vitamin D may play an instrumental role in changing AMH (anti-mullerian hormone) levels - especially in winter - as well as being vital to the proper growth of the uterine lining. There is also some suggestion that a deficiency of Vitamin D may play a role in the development of metabolic syndrome - therefore supplementation for women with PCOS is indicated.

- Prenatal Multivitamin - I recommend a whole food supplement that contains a non-constipating form of Iron. With its easy absorption, it is well tolerated by women experiencing nausea. Contains essential nutrients and folic acid to prepare for and maintain a healthy pregnancy.

- Probiotics* - The World Health Organization (WHO) defines probiotics as "live microorganisms which when administered in adequate amounts confer a health benefit on the host". Probiotics replenish intestinal flora (healthy bacteria) and promote overall digestive and immune health (amongst many other health benefits). The road to health is paved with good intestines. Quality is key with probiotics. I suggest a dairy-free probiotic in specialized capsules so it is able to bypass or resist the harmful effects of stomach acid. A therapeutic dosage of probiotics should be > 10 billion CFU (colony forming units) per day. Lactobacillus acidophilus and Bifidobacterium bifidum are the two strains that best address both small and large intestine. Probiotics work best if the consumer also has regular intake of prebiotics (which feed the probiotics) such as legumes and fruit.

*Be sure to drink filtered water as chlorine (an antibiotic) will destroy the probiotics.

- Folic Acid (folate, B9, 5-MTHF) - Folic acid is used by the body to manufacture DNA, which is required for rapid cell division and organ/tissue formation in the developing baby. Most expectant mothers are aware of the need to supplement with folic acid during pregnancy to prevent neural tube developmental problems in the fetus. To my knowledge, it may be the one and only supplement recommended by most doctors. 5-MTHF is the most bio-available form of folate available and is what I recommend. The liver and intestines must be healthy for proper absorption of folate (again suggesting the importance of probiotics).

- Iron - Whole food easy to digest non-constipating iron supplements are key in my practice, especially for pregnant women diagnosed with iron deficiency. These supplements should also include folate and B12 as deficiencies of these vitamins can cause or further exacerbate an iron deficiency.

Supplementation is especially important for most vegetarians or vegans. Iron helps carry oxygen to every cell in your body. If you are iron deficient, your cells (and your little embryo) may not be receiving the essential life force from the breath you are taking.

- Thyroid Blends - Supplements containing iodine, selenium and tyrosine are known to help support thyroid health and function. It can help manage symptoms of a sluggish thyroid such as: weight gain, feeling tired and cold all the time, hair (including eyebrow) and memory loss, brittle nails/hair and leg swelling, and most importantly, difficulty conceiving and carrying to term. Be sure to rule out thyroid autoimmune Hashimoto's (raised TPO antibodies) before taking iodine as it may cause a flare of immune function resulting in destruction of thyroid tissue. In the case of Hashimoto's autoimmune, thyroiditis supplements for the immune system and inflammation should be emphasized such as Vitamin D, fish oils and probiotics.

A few facts about the thyroid
Dr. Datis Kharrazian

- *The reason it is so important that the thyroid be healthy before conceiving is that the demands on the gland increase when pregnant. If the thyroid is already deficient, then the increased strain during pregnancy may result in inadequate vital functions associated with the thyroid, often ending in miscarriage.*
- *Hypothyroid symptoms: constipation, fatigue, weight gain despite exercise and proper eating*

habits, recurrent pregnancy loss or difficulty conceiving, thinning of hair on scalp and outer ⅓ of eyebrows.
- *Hyperthyroid symptoms: anxiety, palpitations, night sweats.*
- *Vitamin D deficiency has been associated with Hashimoto's and other autoimmune diseases. If you live in a place with a lack of sunlight, are dark skinned, obese, under stress, or your diet is lacking butter, egg yolks, liver and other organ meats, then consider getting tested for a Vitamin D deficiency and supplement accordingly. Salmon species are very high in Vitamin D.*

Quick Tips

Cut back on **gluten, sugar and dairy.** Although not all are gluten-intolerant, the reason we are seeing so much more of it these days is because of over-consumption. I have seen conditions like endometriosis and other inflammatory and allergic conditions improve drastically with the elimination of these foods. I have heard theories linking infertility to celiac disease (an allergy to gluten). These are foods that people are very commonly sensitive or allergic to, which result in fatigue, headaches, bloating, bowel problems, sleep issues, poor concentration, etc. Traditional bread and pasta should be drastically reduced or eliminated, as well as treats and dairy but there are plenty of alternatives that won't leave you feeling deprived. When you decide to replace milk, choose coconut or almond milk. If you are in desperate need of bread (muffins, pastries) and pasta-related alternatives, you are in luck. The gluten-free trend has gained massive traction and options are readily available.

Processed Foods such as deli meats and almost anything

125

that comes packaged, unless otherwise stated, are full of chemicals, with the effects on human health still not completely understood (see Step Seven). The fact is, the plastic many processed foods are packaged in has a chemical within it that is a known endocrine disruptor, meaning it messes with your hormones. Stick to stuff you can pronounce and the colorful foods discussed in the rainbow diet.

Deep Fried Foods are something we know to be unhealthy, so this is not news. Evidence shows that where reproductive and sexual health is concerned, a good rule of thumb is what's bad for your heart is bad for baby-making!

Portions are often the culprit in today's obesity epidemic. We are just eating too much. If our foods are nutritious, smaller portions will fulfill our needs. Obesity is also strongly linked to reproductive health issues such as fertility in both men and women, so pay attention to what your body is telling you. When you are mindful and you eat slowly, you will notice that you probably don't need as much food as you think you do. Stop eating before you get full and never feel like you have to finish everything on your plate. Remember this simple phrase: '*Eating nutritious foods = the need to eat less food*.'

Antioxidants. If you have not heard of this 'fountain of youth' it's time you did. Antioxidants essentially clean up the residues left from the stressful lives we lead and the environmental toxins we come in contact with. Stress and toxins are responsible for a plethora of undesirable things like infertility, aging, skin issues and chronic pain. Antioxidants are found in colorful foods like fruits and vegetables. Therefore, pile your plate high with fresh colorful whole foods and look forward to energy and vibrancy.

Raw Food vs. Cooked Food. There is no conclusive evidence as to which may be better for you. I understand that food is naturally raw in nature, but we were also given the gift of fire. So I think finding a balance of raw and cooked is the way to go. In the true honor of Traditional Chinese Medicine, diet should be individualized for each person depending on their needs. For example, someone with very poor digestion (lots of gas, bloating and loose bowel movements) will not be able to pull nutrients from raw foods and should lean towards soups, stews, juicing, or at the very least, lightly steaming their fruits and veggies. Someone with a lot of 'Heat' who can digest almost anything could benefit greatly from an increased consumption of raw foods. Sometimes raw can mean less processed as is the case with honey or nuts and, in which case, I recommend going that route as more nutrition is retained.

Sugar. Did you know that all the carbs in your diet are turned into sugar during digestion? If it isn't protein, fat or fibre, it will end up as sugar in your body. Carbs are complex sugar, so don't think that just because you haven't had any chocolate today that you're sugar-free.

If you have ovulatory disorders such as Polycystic Ovary Syndrome, this is something you'll want to be mindful of. Too much sugar in any of its forms is shown to overload the system and lead to insulin resistance and possibly diabetes as well as candida and inflammation.

This same overload can lead to ovulatory disturbance. So, cut way down on the carbs. If you do have high blood sugar, increase your fiber intake and try including cinnamon, apple cider vinegar and extra virgin cold-pressed olive oil in your diet to lower your levels. And absolutely *eliminate* sugar's evil cousin, high fructose corn syrup, known in Canada as glucose-fructose.

This man-made sweetener interferes with the body's ability to know when it has had enough food and is stored in the liver as triglycerides and fat. It is chemically similar to alcohol and can damage liver function (which is essential to reproductive health).

When you want something sweet, reach for an organic peach or spread some raw honey or maple syrup on a brown rice cracker. Small changes add up and your body will thank you.

Iron. When your levels are low, eat large amounts of dark green leafy vegetables like chard, kale, dandelion, romaine lettuce, mustard greens and spinach. They are also high in magnesium which is depleted if the body is storing extra estrogens such as with endometriosis, polyps, fibroids, tumors or cysts. If you find your digestion is poor, it is best to cook or steam them using cast iron cookware and to remember to chew thoroughly and relax while eating. I also recommend taking a whole food supplement such as 'Iron Response' by Innate. You will see good results and it's non-constipating.

Eat Organic. Ensure the following 'Dirty Baker's Dozen' foods are always organic: celery, nectarines, apples, grapes, strawberries, peaches, bell peppers, spinach, cherries, pears, lettuce, potatoes and all animal products as these are known to be laden with pesticides. The effects of pesticides and toxins on our health are numerous. When it comes to fertility, especially if there is no other explanation, avoiding the poisons in conventionally-farmed foods can only help. I support the moderate consumption of well-raised and produced animal products if I believe it to be a necessary aspect to your treatment. I encourage you to choose animals that got to run and live a humane life, free of hormones and antibiotics, and were fed a diet of organic foods. Consuming animals who lived full of fear and despair may transfer that negative energy to the person that consumes them. For this reason, I also strongly suggest eliminating the intake of baby animals such as lamb or veal. I suggest you educate yourself on Genetically Modified Organisms (GMO), since we still have very little understanding of what these 'Frankenstein foods' are doing to our health and fertility. For example, many of the GMO seeds produced have genetics built into them so that the seeds produced will never again sprout, called 'terminator' genes. This makes it so that the farmers have to buy new seeds from the company every year to plant their crops, instead of just keeping a few seeds from last year's harvest. If we are eating seeds that are programmed not to reproduce, are these seeds void of essential elements or life forces that *we* require to reproduce? Corn, soy, canola and sugar beets are just a few places to start ensuring you are choosing organic; otherwise, you can guarantee what you are eating is a GMO. Check out the documentary, *GMO OMG*, for a deeper look into this topic.

NOTE: *In Canada, the government has not posed regulation forcing the mandatory labelling of Genetically Modified Foods. The Canadian Biotechnology Action Network reports only four GMO crops are grown in Canada:*

1. corn
2. soy
3. canola
4. sugar beets

Getting Rid of Sugar

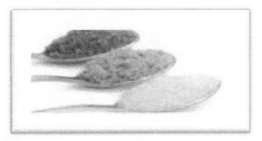

Start by eliminating all unnatural forms of sweeteners (from glucose-fructose and high fructose corn syrup to Aspartame and Splenda), even Stevia in too much quantity (which is a natural plant substance derived from beets and cane), as they are usually a few hundred times sweeter than simple table sugar.

These sweeteners raise your body's desire for obtaining more sweetness, thus creating more profound cravings that are increasingly difficult to suppress. This results in poorer choices (when in the waiting line at Starbucks) and eating greater quantities of carbohydrates.

High fructose corn syrup (glucose-fructose) is different enough in molecular structure that the body's usual feedback mechanisms that tell the brain 'I have had enough sugar' are bypassed, leaving you feeling like you can have more and more and more without being satisfied. Sugar and ALL of its ugly cousins are public enemy #1.

Sugar beets are used to make white table sugar. If you need sugar, please choose cane. As for corn, it is mostly corn used to feed livestock and to produce the popular sweetener glucose-fructose, or high fructose corn syrup. Popcorn and sweet corn are rarely GMO but some say that is changing. Commonly imported GMO foods into Canada include: cottonseed oil, papaya and some squashes such as zucchini and yellow. Contrary to common belief, The Canadian Biotechnology Action Network says there is no GMO wheat in North America, and there are no GMO potatoes or tomatoes anywhere in the world. At the time of publication, the introduction of the first GMO fruit (apple) into Canada is being considered.

True Story

When I was younger, GMO crops were just beginning to be planted on a larger scale. I lived on the prairies of Canada and a farmer that I knew was being threatened legally by the creators of GMO canola. Crops of canola seeds, some GMO and some normal, were being planted close to one another. The GMO seed company tested the nearby neighbouring normal crops and found them to have the patented GMO DNA within. It was believed this must have happened from wind causing cross pollination of the different crops. The farmer had charges brought to him for having planted patented canola without purchasing the seeds from the company in question and his seeds were confiscated. This happened to many farmers until it was apparent to authorities that the real problem might actually be that these Genetically Modified Organisms are now out in the world and we will never be able to recall them due to cross pollination of normal seeds, changing their DNA forever.

Drink Water. Lots of it! Your body thrives when it's well hydrated. It washes away whatever toxins may have built up and revives your cells. Think of it as a shower for your insides. Avoid water that has been stored in plastic bottles, especially the big blue water jugs used on many water coolers as they contain BPA which companies in Canada are not legally allowed to use in children's products, so why is it ok that adults can drink from BPA containers? The damage that the chemicals contained in plastics can leave behind is profound.

If you feel the tap water in your community is of good quality, a filter should suffice or you can let it sit on your counter for a few hours before drinking so that the chlorine has a chance to off-gas. Chlorine is put into our water systems to eliminate living organisms such as bacteria, so consider for a moment what it does to the friendly bacteria in our guts that we need for proper digestion and immune function.

If you live in a city that puts fluoride in your water, please find a clean source that you can purchase for drinking and join the movement to stop this science experiment. The fluoride they put in your water is not the same as that found in toothpaste; it is a waste by-product of the petro-chemical manufacturing industry being marketed and sold back to our governments. The impact of this on our health is yet to be determined.

For those of you that find plain water dull, add lemon or mint to perk it up. Tea is a worthwhile alternative too and many of them have medicinal qualities. Spearmint tea, for example, will help lower androgen levels and ginger aids digestion and helps with bloating and gas. Cut back considerably on coffee and alcohol as both of these are very dehydrating. They have been associated with increased risk of miscarriage and elevated homocysteine levels. And save your beverages for after you are finished eating (especially ice water) so as to allow your digestive juices to do their job without being diluted.

So how much water, you ask? Well, here is a simple formula I like to use; your weight in pounds x 15 = amount of water per day in millilitres (30 ml = 1 oz., 250ml = 1 cup).

Eat Good Fats. Our bodies need fat, it's that simple. The non-fat trend is hopefully on its way out as we are becoming aware that many companies have replaced fats with chemicals that do far more damage than a little fat ever could, and people have replaced their fats (for fear of gaining weight) with sugars, which ironically is the actual cause of our obesity epidemic. Once again, a good rule of thumb is to steer clear of the processed food, only eat organic meats and eliminate dairy completely. If you read the word fat on a package and it's preceded by one like trans saturated, put it down and walk away. Good fats are found in Omega-3 and Omega-6 fatty acids. Omega 3 fats have anti-inflammatory effects and can be found in fish like sardines and salmon or from nuts and seeds. Omega-6 is found in many foods such as avocados, eggs and coconut, whole grain bread and nuts. If you are unable to get adequate intake of good fats through your food, supplements are available, but with so many choices, that shouldn't be necessary.

Food Cures for TCM Patterns

Food cure is the use of foods and herbs intended to elicit a curative effect on the presenting condition. In China, the line between herbs and food is not entirely clear. Herbs are commonly added to dishes for their medicinal qualities rather than taste.

In the chapter on TCM (Step One - Ancient Healing), we talked about the different diagnosis and what they mean for fertility. At the end of the step, you should have listed your top two or three TCM patterns for future reference. You will need these here. Remember, because it is common to exhibit symptoms from more than one pattern, you may find conflicting information below.

Diet & Cleanses

There are thousands of recipes available on websites that are dedicated to healthy and delicious evolution of our diets. If you are missing something, I guarantee there is something just like it that won't cause harm to you.

Also, consider doing an anti-inflammatory dietary cleanse. I recommend Mediclear Plus by Thorne Research. This is an 'elimination-reintroduction' style of cleanse which can help determine foods you may be sensitive or allergic to. I recommend having a healthcare professional follow you throughout your cleanse to ensure safety.

For example, a man may clearly fit into the pattern of Heat but may also show signs of Blood Stasis and Qi Stagnation. Therefore, rank your (or your husband's) presenting TCM patterns in order of importance so that recommendations that are most relevant can be prioritized for implementation.

Lastly, always be mindful of your personal reaction to certain foods. The wrong food can be poison but the right food is medicine.

Yang Deficiency / Cold
Emphasize:
• More onion, leeks, garlic (small amounts), chives, scallions, black beans, Brussels sprouts, sunflower seeds, sesame seeds, walnuts, pine nuts, chestnuts, cashews, fennel, cumin, cherries, dates, shellfish, chicken, beef,

pepper, mustard.

- Animal protein such as lean meats & fish, as well as bone broths and nuts should be a focus.
- Cooked vegetables should also be plentiful to maintain optimal nutrition.
- Omega oils from fat sources such as walnuts, avocados, and fish.
- Warm water.

Avoid:
- Raw uncooked or cold foods (straight from the fridge or freezer) especially in winter.
- Avoid dairy, caffeine, sugars, and processed foods.
- Alcohol, particularly cold beer.

Recipe ideas:
- Shrimp fried in butter, garlic, and pepper
- Bone broth soup with leeks, potatoes, and Brussels sprouts
- Pate - sunflower seeds, sesame seeds, walnuts, mushrooms
- Roast chicken with pepper sage and thyme
- Roasted vegetables with garlic and rosemary
- Rice porridge with cinnamon, nutmeg and a little brown sugar
- Baked squash and root vegetables

Qi Deficiency
Emphasize:
- More chia seeds, congee, oats, quinoa, rice, beef, chicken, herring, lamb, mussels, shrimp, sunflower seeds, sweet potato, watercress and winter squash
- Many smaller meals throughout the day to

raise metabolism
- Minimizing starchy carbohydrates
- Emphasize root vegetables (70% or more cooked, 30% or less raw)
- Animal protein such as lean meats and fish
- Bone broth vegetable soups
- Nuts should be eaten generously
- Room temperature or warm water (weight in lbs. x 15 = ml/day [250ml = 1 cup] recommended)

Avoid:
- Large portions; instead, eat many smaller meals throughout the day.
- Business at meal time. Relax, breathe, enjoy and chew your food.
- Dairy, caffeine, sugars, processed foods.
- Excesses of carbohydrates.
- Alcohol, particularly cold beer.

Recipe ideas:
- Oatmeal with dates, almond milk and maple syrup
- Sunflower seed mushroom and nutritional yeast pate
- Fried peppered shrimp and quinoa
- Steak and sweet potatoes
- Open face sunflower sprouts and seeds with chia, tomato sandwich with lots of pepper
- Soups and stews in general (easy to digest)
- Chicken soup with astragalus
- Forest mushroom stir fry with rice noodle

Blood Deficiency
Emphasize:
- More aduki and kidney beans, beef, beets, bone marrow, eggs, dark leafy greens, apricots, dates, figs, grapes, liver, microalgae,

nettle leaf, avocados, oysters, sardines
- Emphasize root vegetables (75% or more cooked, 25% or less raw)
- Animal protein such as red meats and organs (liver)
- Bone broth vegetable soups and stews
- Nuts and whole grains should be eaten generously
- Room temperature or warm water (weight in lbs. x 15 = ml/day [250ml = 1 cup] recommended)

Avoid:
- Dairy, caffeine, sugars, processed foods.
- Excessive legume intake.

Recipe ideas:
- Hard boiled eggs with avocados
- Beef bone broth and root vegetable soup
- Liver and onions
- Nuts and dates
- Oil and vinegar fried spinach
- Roasted root vegetables (beets & yams) with rosemary and dill

Heat
Emphasize:
- More fruit, sprouts, mung beans, seaweed, lettuce, cucumber, radish, celery, asparagus, chard, spinach, bok choy, cauliflower, sweet corn, zucchini, apple, asian pears, watermelon, citrus, fish and nuts.
- 50-75% of your food intake should consist of colorful (particularly green) vegetables (50% raw, 50% cooked).
- Cook lightly and include plenty of raw food.
- Fresh vegetable juice and smoothies are recommended.

- Drink lots of room temperature or cool water as dehydration is often an issue (weight in lbs. x 15 = ml/day [250ml = 1 cup] recommended).
- Eat more bitter foods such as endive and dandelion greens.
- Relax, breathe, enjoy and chew your food.

Avoid:
- spicy, processed, and greasy foods, dairy, alcohol, coffee, garlic, lamb, beef, shellfish, curries, ginger, cinnamon, pepper.
- Eating 'on the go' or skipping meals.
- Alcohol.

Recipe ideas:
- Fresh fruit and veggie smoothies
- Leafy salads with dandelion greens, cucumbers and sprouts
- Miso soup with plenty of seaweed and tofu
- Watermelon watermelon watermelon - particularly in summer months
- Wild rice and barley with mung beans, apples and shredded almonds
- Baked white fish with lemon and sweet corn
- Avocados with a dash of salt
- Water with mint leaves
- Mung bean soup
- Mung bean vermicelli with scallops
- Green papaya salad with cilantro, sesame oil and lime

Dampness & Phlegm
Emphasize:
- More legumes, black pepper, seaweeds, lean meats, fish, bone broths
- Lightly cooked vegetables (65% cooked 35% raw).

- Reduce the amount of food eaten at one sitting, instead eat many smaller meals throughout the day.
- Relaxation and thorough chewing of food.
- More soups and stews will be easier to digest and should be a focus. Add flavours that are aromatic to assist with digestion: cardamom, cinnamon, ginger, cloves, turmeric, rosemary, parsley, marjoram, tarragon.
- Drink lots of room temperature water (weight in lbs. x 15 = ml/day recommended).
- Start each meal by taking a few deep breaths to smell your food, allow the saliva to build up in your mouth; it is full of the digestive enzymes ready to break down your meal. Do not drink any water just before eating; sip on water throughout your meal instead.

Avoid:
- Dairy - all types, especially milk, ice cream, soft cheeses, yogurt.
- Deep fried food.
- Smoothies, fruit juices.
- Soft nuts - peanuts, cashews, pistachios.
- Sugar and all sweet foods (baked goods, desserts, dried fruits).
- Limit raw food intake.
- Alcohol - all types.
- Large meal portions.
- Bananas and all other tropical fruits.
- Sticky grains; oatmeal, wheat, spelt, rye, millet.

Recipe ideas:
- Spaghetti squash with lentils and stir fried mushrooms and onions
- BBQ vinegar-marinated asparagus with black pepper

- Celery and hummus
- Lettuce wraps with white beans and white fish
- Fried peppered shrimp and quinoa
- Tomato purple cabbage caraway soup
- Roasted chicken with lemon, tarragon and black pepper
- Spanish paella with chorizo sausage, chicken and prawns (oregano, bay leaf, paprika, saffron, pepper, garlic, onions, chili, parsley)
- Breakfast frittata with mushrooms, spinach, oregano, olives, artichoke

Blood Stasis

Emphasize:
- More turmeric, scallions, nutmeg, chives, garlic, vinegar, basil, ginger, chestnuts, rosemary, cayenne, pomegranate, gobo, lotus root, cabbage, soybean, Jew's ear, corn, prawn, squid.
- 50-75% of food intake should consist of colorful (particularly green) vegetables (50% raw, 50% cooked).
- Fish and nuts as primary sources of protein.
- A little spicy food can be beneficial but caution if there are prominent Heat signs.
- Stay well hydrated. Room temperature water (weight in lbs. x 15 = ml/day [250ml = 1 cup] recommended).

Avoid:
- Dairy, sugar, processed foods.
- Excessive sour-flavoured foods.
- Deep fried greasy food and saturated fats.
- Large portions.
- Excessive amounts of spicy foods if signs of Heat are present (see above).

Recipe ideas:
- Roasted onions, garlic and yam with rosemary and cayenne
- Chicken rice noodle soup with scallions chives and ginger
- Pickled jalapenos or banana peppers
- Spicy curried eggplant
- Peppered roasted chestnuts
- Korean short ribs and kimchi
- Stir fried gobo and lotus root with sesame oil and tamari
- Seafood curry soup

Qi Stagnation
Emphasize:
- More green apples, peppermint and spearmint, orange peel tea, rosemary, scallions, onion, fennel, anise, dill, mustard and dandelion greens, basil, nutmeg, marjoram, elder flowers, radish and its leaves, taro and turnip.
- 50-75% of food intake should consist of colorful (particularly green) vegetables (50% raw, 50% cooked).
- Fish and nuts as a primary protein source.
- Staying hydrated. Drink lots of room temperature or slightly cool water (weight in lbs. x 15 = ml/day [250ml = 1 cup] recommended).
- Relax, breathe, enjoy and chew your food.

Avoid:
- Excessive sour foods like vinegar, pickles.
- Alcohol.
- Dairy, caffeine, sugars, processed foods.
- Too many comfort foods (carbohydrates) to ease emotional stagnation will lead to digestive upset (gas, bloating).

- Business at meal time. Relax, breathe, enjoy and chew your food.

Recipe ideas:
- Mustard greens salad with peppermint and radish
- Pickled fennel
- Green apples and pistachios
- Fried radish leaves and onions in vinegar and oil with dill
- Pickled lotus root with yuzu zest

Yin Deficiency
Emphasize:
- More fish, root vegetables, seeds, nuts (walnuts), eggs, dark leafy greens, dates, liver, some fatty cuts of meat, and bone marrow.
- Microalgae like chlorella, spirulina and wild blue-green.
- Omega oils from fat sources such as evening primrose, avocados, and fish.
- Slightly larger meal portions or include soup with each meal.
- Cook lightly and include plenty of raw food.
- Fresh vegetable juice and smoothies are recommended.
- Staying hydrated. Drink lots of room temperature or cool water (weight in lbs. x 15 = ml/day [250ml = 1 cup] recommended).
- Relax, breathe, enjoy and chew your food.

Avoid:
- Spicy food, legumes, coffee, alcohol, sugars, shellfish and processed foods, especially in summer and fall.
- Alcohol.
- Eating 'on the go' or skipping meals.

Recipe ideas:
- Fruit and leafy green smoothies with maple syrup and banana
- Fish dishes with coconut milk
- Omelette with mushrooms and black beans
- Asparagus and egg salads with sesame seeds
- Tacos made with kidney beans and topped with a small amount of cheese
- Baked Potato stuffed with tofu, soy sauce (Braggs) and sesame seeds
- Pork and apple dishes
- Miso soup with udon noodles tofu and seaweed
- Bone broth soup with lotus root, goji berries and pine nuts
- Oatmeal with molasses, goji berries, raisins and cinnamon

To detoxify the liver and restore hormonal balance, eat cruciferous vegetables: broccoli, Brussels sprouts, cabbage, collards, cauliflower, kale, kohlrabi, mustard greens, rapeseed and root vegetables such as turnips and rutabagas.

A lot of the time when people hear the word diet, they cringe. In our society, 'diets' have become synonymous with depriving oneself or feeling guilty and that shouldn't be the case. Food is your friend and it is a valuable tool to nourish your body and give it what it needs to operate at maximum capacity. Learn what foods are right for you and you will be filled with gratitude for the strength and vitality they give you.

Story
Andrea H.

I stopped using hormonal birth control in August 2011 and began having irregular cycles. All of my initial bloodwork and testing was normal so there was no obvious cause for this and we were referred to PCRM. We met with an RE at PCRM in July 2012, Clomid was prescribed and I began acupuncture with a local practitioner.

From April – October 2012 - I was taking Visalus meal replacements which are soy-based. The acupuncturist suggested possibly quitting this due to the soy content and I decided to do this. I wasn't noticing many changes from my acupuncture appointments; in fact my cycles seemed to be more unregulated, regularly ending in 10 days of Provera.

A friend recommended Dr. Spence Pentland and I began seeing him once a week around the time of my 2nd Clomid cycle in November 2012. In December, we added Inositol (3000 mg/day). Throughout this time, I was taking Clomid and ovulated somewhat regularly but had a slower response the 3rd time on 50mg.

I saw Spence for about a year. He was so encouraging throughout the whole process. He supported whatever decisions we made, including pursuing treatment with western medicine but always offered complementary TCM options and alternatives.

In January 2013, we added Chinese Herbs (2/day), EPA (2/day) and Vitamin D to my daily regime and limited gluten, dairy, caffeine, soy and alcohol from my diet. As a result, I saw more regular menstrual cycles with unmedicated ovulation, better digestion and increased energy.

We attempted our 4th cycle of Clomid (increasing the dose to 100mg and did our first IUI) in February 2013 and became pregnant but this pregnancy ended in miscarriage at 9 weeks.

We took a break for April and then in May got back to all of the above. My husband took Carnityl and EPA at this time too. We tried another Clomid/IUI cycle in June 2013 and again became pregnant but it was a chemical pregnancy ending at 4 1/2 weeks.

We had repeat loss testing and again everything was normal. We decided to see a different RE for another opinion on the next steps, enjoy the summer and get 'healthy' in the meantime while continuing to see Dr. Pentland weekly. I continued with the gluten/dairy free diet, limited caffeine and alcohol, took the herbs and supplements, adding CoQ10 and baby aspirin and focusing on a high protein/low carb eating. During this time period, I also began running 3x/week. My husband continued to take Carnityl, EPA and added CoQ10 as well. He had 'normal' sperm analysis but his results were actually very borderline. He was quite concerned with his counts during our IUI's. We can't help but think the supplements were useful.

Without drugs or IUI, I got my 3rd positive pregnancy test in September 2013. I continued with weekly acupuncture, aspirin and took progesterone supplements to help maintain the pregnancy. I'm due in May 2014.

While I know it will be worth it, the process of making a baby wasn't an easy one. I went through all the emotions, I think. I often was quite bitter and upset, especially with friends that seemed to take their fertility/kids for granted and especially after my losses. I was often mostly upset at not ovulating and therefore even having a chance. With each new treatment, I had renewed hope. With each pregnancy I was anxious about loss again. It was oftentimes hard on my marriage as well. Trying to conceive became very controlled and regimented, and it stole a lot of our intimacy. I think in the end it will make us stronger but we aren't there yet since we are still dealing with pregnancy hormones. I do really appreciate being pregnant though, and haven't had much to complain about. I'm not sure if I've just had a relatively easy pregnancy or if others that didn't have to work as hard for it just take it for granted and complain about it. I'm guessing I'll feel this way about our baby as well.

Owen Zachary was joyfully welcomed on May 25th at 2:59pm. He was 53 cm. and a whopping 9 lbs. 4oz. after an unplanned C-section. Everyone is doing well.

Chapter Task:

List three improvements to your diet that you will start to implement today:

1. _____

2. _____

3. _____

Write down any questions you still have about diet:

_____

_____

_____

_____

Now go and find answers to these questions!

Step Six

Get Moving

What to do and How to Start

"An early-morning walk is a blessing for the whole day."
~Henry David Thoreau

D efinition of exercise: *any bodily activity that enhances or maintains physical fitness and overall health and wellness. It is performed for various reasons including strengthening muscles and the cardiovascular system, honing athletic skills, weight loss or maintenance, as well as for the purpose of enjoyment.*

Some people hear the word exercise and wince, but that doesn't have to be the case. Like diet, different exercise plans work for different people and the key to finding what is right for you is that it be something you enjoy.

Finding something you like to do that also happens to be exercise should not be a problem. There are as many choices these days as there are types of people. What about a Zumba class? Or kick boxing? Martial Arts? Pole dancing? Rock climbing? A team sport like volleyball or soccer maybe? You could go kayaking or take a surf trip or try fencing if you're feeling adventurous.

There are no limits to the possibilities for fun with fitness and the benefits of exercise are no secret. Expect to lower your body fat, increase energy and muscle mass, reduce stress, improve your circulation, better sleep, lower blood pressure and feel an overall sense of well-being and confidence. And let's not forget the most important benefit of all - with increased health comes increased fertility. So if you're serious about starting a family, some form of exercise is a must.

The goal is to maintain a healthy body weight and steer away from being too thin or keeping up with an exercise regime that may be too strenuous. If your body is repairing muscles that are being used excessively, it will have less energy to devote to reproductive health.

If your weight is too low or too high, it will affect hormonal balance and ovulation. Women that are underweight will often have a lack of estrogen which can cause menstruation to be irregular or cease all together, so in spite of the cultural messages we see portrayed in magazines nowadays, there is such a thing as too thin.

If you find yourself overweight due to a lack of exercise but you're not sure where to start, take a walk. Aerobic exercise is key for weight loss and is considered anything that involves performing continuous movements, in your specific aerobic target heart range, with large muscle groups such as your legs, for 20 minutes or more. Cycling, swimming, rowing, walking, dancing or jogging are just a few examples of aerobic exercise. Low-intensity sessions that last at least 30-45 minutes are ideal for weight loss.

There's no need for a gym membership or athletic prowess, it can be as simple as four brisk, half-hour walks a week to get your heart pumping and increase circulation; something that strongly assists with increased fertility.

In conjunction with addressing physical activity, Traditional Chinese Medicine (TCM) emphasizes the importance of cultivating willpower to overcome conditions such as overeating, laziness, and obesity. Acupuncture and Chinese herbal medicine supplement the systems necessary for being proactive in one's life and making healthy choices for mind and body. With time, discipline and simple small commitments, the trajectory of your entire life can change. A healthy life is a fulfilling life and everyone deserves that.

Elements to consider when attempting to manifest a holistic exercise regime are: Agility, Flexibility, Strength, Speed, Balance, Stamina, Coordination and Endurance.

Exercise Recommendations for Specific Reproductive Challenges

Unexplained Infertility: Yoga is a balanced form of exercise that often has a meditative aspect to it that will allow you to get in touch with yourself. Oftentimes unexplained infertility can be attributed to stress and taking the time to breathe in combination with challenging poses will release this stress and clue you in to what's going on with your body and spirit.

Advanced Maternal Age: The inevitabilities of time and possibly neglect take their toll on our bodies and it is important to address typical conditions and symptoms such as poor circulation and decreased muscle tone specifically. Improving blood flow to reproductive organs can often be the solution to age-related fertility hold-ups so cardiovascular activity is recommended as it gets the blood pumping where it needs to. Also, since muscle tone decreases with age, a fitness routine that includes moderate weight lifting would be beneficial to women over thirty-five.

Polycystic Ovary Syndrome: A focus on muscle building is important for women with PCOS. Weight-bearing exercise will reduce insulin resistance, which will help reverse the hormonal imbalance that is causing the problems associated with PCOS. Fat-burning aerobic exercise should be another goal. A well-rounded routine including lunges, squats, bicep curls and aerobic activity as discussed above will help reduce high estrogen and testosterone levels thus improving your chances of ovulation and conception.

FAT FACTS

"A person generally gains fat-related weight by increasing food consumption, becoming physically inactive, or both. When energy (food) intake exceeds energy expenditure (movement), the body stores the excess as fat." Despite this widely accepted statement being logical, it is shortsighted and oversimplified. It should be emphasized that it is the over-consumption of the 'wrong foods' that is causing the storage of excess fats, even when energy expenditure exceeds food energy (caloric) intake.

Stress and Anxiety: Some people with busy lives and high stress levels may take comfort in the rhythmic movement of Tai Chi or yoga. For others, a rigorous run or downhill skiing are the way to release stress. In this case, I would say, if it feels good, do it!

Below is a study prepared by The Practice Committee of the American Society for Reproductive Medicine in Birmingham, Alabama and published in Fertility and Sterility, Volume 90 in November of 2008:

This Educational Bulletin describes the effect of obesity on reproduction and concluded from an analysis of over 95 peer-reviewed research studies pertaining to obesity and fertility. National Institutes of Health (NIH) defines obesity in relation to body mass index (BMI); overweight was defined as a BMI between 25 and 29.9, obesity as a BMI 30.

In my practice, I most certainly see a negative correlation between obesity and fertility success. It is something I counsel on being of primary importance when a woman of BMI greater than 25 is trying to fall pregnant.

Myo-inositol (a dietary supplement) has been shown to restore regular ovulation, lower insulin, and decrease androgens.

Sources:
("Myo-inositol: true progress in the treatment of polycystic ovary syndrome and ovulation induction".
M. GALLETTA, et al - Reproductive Medicine Unit, Hera Association, Catania (Italy) - *Department of Obstetrics and Gynaecology, Messina University (Italy) - **Palm Beach Center for Reproductive Medicine, Wellington, FL (USA). European Review for Medical and Pharmacological Sciences - 2011; 15: 1212-1214)

Summary
- Obesity is associated with menstrual dysfunction (irregular ovulation and cycles), decreased fertility and increased risk of miscarriages.
- Obesity decreases fertility, even in women that are ovulating regularly.
- Obesity increases the risks of pregnancy and postpartum complications.
- Obesity is associated with abnormal semen parameters and may adversely affect male fertility.

- Preconceptual counseling for obese women should address the medical, pregnancy and postpartum consequences of obesity and its longer-term implications for offspring.
- Lifestyle changes involving a diet and exercise program are the first-line treatment for obesity.

The impact of obesity on reproductive function can be attributed primarily to hormonal imbalances. Excessive abdominal weight is associated with increased insulin levels, which result in increased male hormone (androgen) levels. Fat tissue transforms much of these androgens into estrogen which becomes chronically elevated causing an imbalanced menstrual cycle and pre/post natal abnormalities listed above.

Story
Raj D.

I've always wanted to be a mom. I always took for granted that I would be a mom. Today, I am the mother of a 5 year-old girl – the little love of my life but having her was quite the journey...and worth every little heartache along the way.

When I got married at almost 33 years old, I was on methotrexate, a drug I needed to treat rheumatoid arthritis which I had been diagnosed with at the age of 16. It's a cancer drug and an ingredient in the morning-after-pill and had to be out of my system before I could even try to get pregnant or risk miscarriage or fetal abnormalities. My rheumatologist put me on a steroid called prednisone, I saw a genetic counselor, and I went on a cleanse to rid my body of toxins. I had the go-ahead in the fall of 2004.

The prednisone caused me to gain weight but it was a miracle drug in terms of treating my arthritis. Unfortunately, the weight I gained was in my face and around my belly and I was always being asked if I was pregnant, but month after disappointing month, I was not.

By September of 2005, I had visited my family doctor and started undergoing the usual battery of tests to determine the cause of my fertility issues. Given my age and the fact that I had been trying to get pregnant for almost a year, I was referred to the U.B.C. Fertility Clinic where I was given Clomid and had three IUIs. After the third attempt to get pregnant with IUI, it was decided that I would try IVF. Despite increasing doses of fertility medications, IVF was not working and my cycle was cancelled. Only 3 or 4 follicles grew and reduced my chances of a successful pregnancy.

That cycle was particularly difficult as I had been trying to be as natural as possible and was not on any drugs to control my arthritis. I had fractured my ankle as well and tried not to take painkillers, and on the way home from one appointment where I was told the cycle wasn't working, I got into a car accident. That was probably one of the worst days of my life. The day the fertility specialist told me that my cycle would be cancelled was another one of those days. No one batted an eyelash when I said I had arthritis but when reviewing my results, the fertility specialist told me that my arthritis had possibly attacked my ovaries and that she would have to research the effects of arthritis on fertility. Huh? I thought. I didn't know one had anything to do with the other. My rheumatologist had talked about how women with arthritis generally had fewer children due to their health but didn't say anything about it affecting fertility. I had taken myself off of drugs and went through considerable pain to try to get pregnant, and unknowingly, I may have caused the infertility? I was beyond upset and I was certainly not going to go back.

I then tried IVF again hoping for a better outcome. At the IVF clinic, I learned about acupuncture and I decided to explore how the mind helps the body to get healthy and to get pregnant. I met Dr. Spence Pentland and was immediately at ease in his care. Not one to nap or fall asleep anywhere other than in a bedroom at night, I found myself to get so relaxed with him that I could hear myself snoring and didn't even care that he could too. Spence advised me about Chinese medicine. He gave me magic potions to drink which cured some circulation issues because I used to be cold all the time and to this day, that no longer happens. Despite Spence's care and attention over two visits a week and into my next IVF cycle, the results were similar. I took a little time off, continued to get acupuncture and began to take Mediclear. The next IVF cycle yielded more follicles, but still not enough to proceed. I'd had two cancelled cycles over a period of a year despite the maximum dosages of IVF drugs. This time, I was told that I was unable to get pregnant with my own eggs but I could try with donor eggs. I was crushed.

Around the same time, my friend, a family physician, told me that a patient of hers had seen an IVF doctor by the name of Dr. Z in San Francisco. Similar to me, her patient had not responded to IVF treatments here but she was pregnant and had frozen embryos through her treatments there. I decided to give it a shot.

My first appointment was a telephone consultation. I had sent Dr. Z my file and clearly, he had read it. One of the first things he asked me was if I had ever been on a drug called Humira for my arthritis but I hadn't. He explained to me that he specialized in auto-immune issues related to infertility. He was worried about my BMI. since I had gained 30 pounds due to the steroids I had been using to treat my arthritis. Dr. Zouves suggested that I try to lose weight, get started on Humira, and call him if and when I was interested in pursuing a cycle under his guidance.

I underwent expensive and extensive tests prior to

commencing an IVF cycle. The staff at the San Francisco Fertility Centre were amazingly helpful and informative. I encountered some resistance at various medical facilities here as some of the tests were only performed once a few miscarriages had taken place and I hadn't even managed to get pregnant yet. Regardless, a few people broke some bureaucratic rules for me. I had lost 20 pounds, I was seeing Spence for acupuncture and in March 2008, I flew to San Francisco to start my IVF cycle. There probably wasn't that much difference in the follicle result with Dr. Z, however, he was always reassuring and my cycle was not going to be cancelled with 3 or 4 follicles. It only takes one embryo to get pregnant I was told. In the end, it was all I had and it was enough. Dr. Z himself called to congratulate me. His clinic had always made me feel like a person, not a statistic.

The Dr. Z protocol did not end there though. I was giving myself progesterone injections and I was on Humira until I was 3 months along. I continued to see Spence until that time as well and I saw him again during the last few weeks of my pregnancy when my daughter was breech and it was suggested that she manually be turned (something I refused to do).

My daughter, Mahla, never did turn around. She was delivered via C-section on December 18, 2008. A perfect, beautiful bundle of joy. I couldn't take my eyes off her then and I still can't. I am incredibly lucky. I believed in her and in myself and the team of professionals I was fortunate enough to work with, and made my little dream come true.

Chapter Task:

List three types of physical activity you will begin to incorporate into your life this week (i.e. stretching, aerobic walking, lunges):

1. _____

2. _____

3. _____

Write down any questions you still have about physical activity:

_____

_____

_____

_____

Now go and find answers to these questions!

Step Seven

Toxin Awareness

What to avoid when you're trying to conceive

"The essence of strategy is knowing what not to do."
~Michael Porter

We've talked a lot about what *to* do to increase your chances of pregnancy but if you're doing everything right and conception is still stalled, you might want to look at what *not* to do.

This chapter is of particular importance for women of advanced maternal age, with unexplained infertility, endometriosis, fibroids, cysts or polyps and for men since sperm are highly sensitive.

Environmental toxins are a very passionate topic in my life. My desire to create awareness through strong emphasis on the negative impacts of these substances and products may, at times, create fear and the feeling that major damage has already been done. This could then be followed by a sense of despair, resentment and not knowing what to do. I apologize if any version of this is your experience, but to some degree if it is, I have done my job! That said, beginning the process of reversing damage caused by toxins is simply a matter of starting to incorporate choices that lead to a cleaner, less toxic personal environment. Start today, it's easier than you think.

No one is immune to the health ailments that are being caused by environmental factors and educating yourself is key not only for conception, but also for parenting. Health challenges like Autism and cancers are rising steadily for kids and have been linked to common pesticides. Learn as much as you can and avoid what you can.

There are over 80,000 manmade chemicals existing in the marketplace today. Most have been introduced since the end of World War II when the petro-chemical companies no longer had a market for chemical weapons, so they found uses for their products in the form of home and agricultural pesticides and fertilizers, food preservatives, household cleaners and personal care products.

Current estimates place the existence of over 200 of these industrially produced chemicals in the human body at any given time. The time when a human is at greatest risk of the effects of these toxins is during fetal development, hence the added relevance for this book. Many of these chemicals are known toxins that disrupt hormonal balance and are contributing factors in infertility, PMS, irregular menstrual cycles, polycystic ovary syndrome, endometriosis, premature ovarian failure, recurrent pregnancy loss, anxiety and cancer of all kinds.

I recently heard a statistic that one half of all Americans will have cancer at some point in their life. It is time to start taking a hard look at the causes, instead of pouring all available money into treatments.

The following table is a list of toxic chemical ingredients commonly found in cosmetic and beauty products (look for on product label), what they are typically used for and the negative effects they have on humans.

Chemical	Use	Effects
BHA, BHT	• Moisturizers • Makeup	• Interfere with hormone function • May cause cancer
Coal tar dyes or FD&C Colors (P-PHENYL-ENEDIAMINE, or colors identified as 'C.I.' followed by 5 digits)	• Hair dyes • Products with coloring	• Skin sensitivities • Contaminated with heavy metals • Toxic to the brain • Deplete oxygen • Cause cancer
CYCLOMETHICONE, SILOXANES	• Moisturizers • Makeup • Hair products	• Interfere with hormone function • Cause liver damage
DEA, MEA, TEA	• Creamy and foaming products (shampoo, moisturizers, etc.)	• Forms cancer causing nitrosamines • Accumulates in body organs and the brain • Contact dermatitis
PHTHALATES (DIBUTYL)	• Usually not listed on labels • Nail products • Perfumes • Makeup • Many other personal care products • Pesticides • Plastics	• Toxic to reproduction • Reduced sperm counts • Interfere with hormone function • Birth defects • Liver/kidney damage • Early breast development in girls and boys
Formaldehyde-releasing preservatives (DMDM HYDANTOIN, DIAZOLIDINYL, UREA, IMIDAZOLIDINYL UREA, METHENAMINE, QUARTERNIUM-15)	• Widely used in hair products Moisturizers	• Cause cancer • Joint pain • Allergies • Depression • Headaches • Chest pain • Chronic fatigue • Insomnia • Dizziness

Chemical	Use	Effects
PARABENS (METHYL, BUTYL, ETHYL, PROPYL)	• Not always labeled • Makeup • Moisturizers • Deodorants • Lubricants • Preservatives	• Interfere with hormone function • Associated with breast cancer • Male infertility • Early puberty
PARFUM or FRAGRANCE	• Most products with scent • Often the last ingredient listed • May be in unscented	• Allergies and asthma • Linked to cancer • Neurotoxicity
PEG (POLYETHYLENE GLYCOL)	• Many types of personal care products • Sunscreen • Conditioners • Moisturizers • Deodorants • Often contaminated with Dioxin	• May cause cancer • If containing dioxins cause multiple reproductive issues including miscarriages and sperm abnormalities amongst others.
PETROLATUM	• Hair & skin care products • Lip balm • Lip stick	•Often contaminated with cancer causing impurities
SODIUM LAURETH SULFATE (SLES), SODIUM LAURYL SULFATE (SLS)	• 90% of personal care products that foam contain SLES and/or SLS • Soap • Shampoo • Bubble bath • Toothpaste	• May cause cancer • Liver damage • Depression • Laboured breathing • Diarrhea • Eye damage • Skin irritation

Chemical	• Use	• Effects
TRICLOSAN	• Antibacterial products • Toothpaste • Soaps • Hand sanitizers • Pesticide	• Interfere with hormone function • Contribute to 'antibiotic resistant' bacteria • May cause cancer
BENZOYL PEROXIDE	• Acne products	• Tumor promoter • Mutagen; cellular DNA damage • Eye, skin, respiratory irritant
Sunscreen Chemicals (AVOBENZONE, BENSPHENONE, ETHOXYCINNAMATE, PABA)	• Sunscreen	• Male infertility (Bensphenone) • Damage to cellular DNA • May lead to cancer • Free radical generators

Sources;

- *davidsuzuki.org*
- *thehealthylivinglounge.com*
- *earthsave.org*
- *tlc.howstuffworks.com*
- *safecosmetics.org*
- *nrdc.org*

Beauty or Beast?

Sixty percent of what goes *on* our bodies gets *in* our bodies so researching skin care and beauty products is hugely important. Fortunately there are now companies that are becoming more responsible.

Read the ingredient list on everything you buy and if there isn't one, know that this is a very bad sign! Fortunately there are more and more companies getting on board with healthy alternatives. By doing your homework and buying products that don't contain harmful ingredients, we increase the demand for them. Even though many cosmetics and beauty companies have been selling us products that can have fatal effects for many years, the consumer is in charge. Don't buy it and they won't sell it. It's time for a beauty revolution!

Here are some more examples of what to look for and avoid:

> *Deodorant and antiperspirant*: Toxic ingredients like parabens, Aluminum, Propylene Glycol, TEA & DEA have all been linked to breast cancer, Alzheimer's disease, kidney and liver failure. As this has become more well known, many great alternatives have popped up. Supply and demand is a powerful tool.

> *Fragrance:* This includes everything from perfume to shampoo to laundry soap to hand cream, air fresheners, dryer sheets and anything else that is scented. When you see the word 'fragrance' on a label it is a synonym for 'chemical compound producing scent' and by law does not have to be identified. Another dirty little trick is that the word 'unscented' can also be used to describe a number of chemicals. Many of which are linked to cancer, reproductive toxicity, hormone disruption and allergies. Opt for essential oils and natural products for a healthier you.

> *Talc:* The primary ingredient in powder not only for you but for your baby's bottom, it is classified as a carcinogen by the International Agency for Research on Cancer if it contains asbestiform fibers, which it often does, but is unregulated so they don't have to tell you that.

> *Tampons:* Have you heard of toxic shock syndrome? Tampons do come with a warning that

'toxic shock syndrome' is a possibility but how many women know what that means? Basically, a tampon causes micro tears in the vaginal walls which allow whatever is in that tampon to penetrate. Tampons have been rumoured to contain asbestos, bleaching agents, dioxins (which refer to numerous chemicals) and rayon fibers, made of wood pulp that has been bleached. While the FDA denies this, again, do your research and if there is an alternative (like a sea sponge or a cup) that you are comfortable with, give it a try.

Toothpaste: Fluoride, like we talked about with regard to water, though banned in many countries, still abides in many toothpastes here and is linked to reproductive problems in men, brain damage, decreased thyroid function and early puberty. Ingredients like detergent, formaldehyde, paraffin, titanium dioxide and saccharin can also be found in many brands and the side effects of these chemicals are nothing to smile about. Again. There are responsible brands out there now but if you want a safe and inexpensive alternative, baking soda and water works well or you can make your own paste using essential oils.

Nail Polish: The majority of nail polish contains chemicals like Dibutyl phthalate, Formaldehyde and Toluene, which are linked to cancer, kidney failure, respiratory problems and developmental issues as it is transferred through breast milk. Read more about nail polish at DavidSuzuki.org (Queen of Green blog).

Some brands that have your best interests and the ingredients to back it up:
- Aveda
- Osmosis

163

- Lush
- Nourish Organic
- Tom's
- Taslie

For nail polish:
- Honeybee Garden
- Piggy Paint
- Suncoat.

These will all come off with rubbing alcohol.

*Coconut oil, avocado, and raw honey are great moisturizers for skin and hair and perfectly safe to consume. This is a good thing to keep in mind with babies and young kids since they are in close contact with you and may suckle your fingers, giving you delightful open mouth kisses, etc.

Lab tests commissioned by the Campaign for Safe Cosmetics found a total of 38 chemicals not listed on the labels in 17 name brand fragrances.

We are All in this Together...

Everything is connected. A great example of this can be seen in Theo Colborn's book, *Our Stolen Future*, in which he tells the tale of a single PCB molecule (a cancer causing chemical found in coolants and banned in 1979) travelling from a factory in Texas to the bottom of a Great Lake, to a Polar bear in Norway twenty years later.

Drastic changes in the reproductive health, patterns and

behaviors of species living around heavily polluted areas (sewage, garbage, agricultural and pharmaceutical run off, PCB's, etc.) is no secret and we are adding more chemicals each day. We are told by industry leaders and government that all are individually tested but the real danger, and something that can never be studied in totality, is how these chemicals interact when they are in our water, food and air.

But You're on Your Own...

The food and drug industry is big business and you really have to look out for yourself. Be sure to read labels and go organic when possible. Some women have had success by going vegan but if that seems too extreme, try your best to eat only free-range, organic fed animal products. When you can buy locally, by all means do. Not only are you getting fresher, less processed food, you are supporting the local economy and sending a message to the large corporations that care more about their bottom line than your health.

Remember, just say no to:

- Non-organic animal products (i.e., meat, eggs and dairy)
- Non-organic foods due to pesticide use and genetic modification (see Step Five)
- Water that has been stored in a plastic container and possibly exposed to temperature extremes
- Cleaning agents that contain fragrance (laundry, body, hair, dish, household)
- Dryer sheets and fabric softeners
- Cosmetic lines that are not completely transparent about their ingredients
- Food that has been microwaved -- especially in plastic containers
- Artificial and manmade sweeteners (see Step Five)

165

- Domestic home and garden pesticides
- Canned foods (unless specified non-BPA lining)
- Phthalates (used in cosmetics and to soften plastic)
- For new homes and office building environments (full of paint, new furniture and flooring, mattresses, photocopiers, etc.) please consider purchasing an air filtration system* that reduces Volatile Organic Compounds, like the one we use at our clinic.

*(http://www.zandair.com - used in IVF laboratory settings to protect embryos from harmful volatile organic compounds)

NOTE: *Volatile Organic Compounds (VOC) are very useful in the natural world. Humans, animals and plants all use subtle VOC scents to communicate with one another on instinctual levels but manmade VOC's are very hazardous to human health. Respiratory, allergic and immune problems are amongst the primary concerns, especially in infants and children. Perfumes and scents of synthetic nature, flooring, paint, furniture, solvents, cleaners, smoke, vehicle exhaust, by-products of plastic and synthetic fiber manufacturing, adhesives (and removers), bed mattresses, dry cleaning, office equipment off gassing and ceiling tiles all emit toxic Volatile Organic Compounds, and their effects to our reproductive health are largely unknown.*

Some Really, Really Bad Guys

Here's a list of common substances that have been shown to have estrogen-mimicking and other endocrine-hormonal disruptive effects. Aptly named, they are collectively known as 'endocrine disruptors'.

Dioxins are by-products of manufacturing chlorine. They are formed during combustion and during the production of chemical compounds containing chlorine, such as pesticides and PCBs. The production and use of some chlorinated chemicals, bleaching of paper and waste incineration, including the uncontrolled burning of residential waste, are the major sources of dioxins. *Reproductive effects*, including decreased sperm production, decreased testis weight, decreased testosterone levels, delayed puberty and endometriosis have been observed in laboratory animals.

Q & A about Cosmetics

Q: Dr. Pentland, can you look at the ingredient list of my skincare creams and tell me if they are safe when I am trying to conceive or pregnant?

A: At first glance, there are still many ingredients I would have to research to know for sure what they are, but that is just looking at the research that exists on each individual ingredient. Studying all possible combinations of various chemicals and their impact on human (reproductive) health is something scientists believe to be closer to science fiction then ever being a reality. For me, the simpler the better, especially for people with sensitive skin. I believe women put themselves in the hands of the creator of the product mixed with a little luck/hope when personal care products are used. All I know is that the cosmetic industry is not regulated, so they do not even have to disclose contaminants or what makes up the product fragrance. If you didn't make it yourself, you really have no way of knowing. I do not think anyone can answer your question, to be quite honest. If it is fine on your skin, and you are as sensitive as you are, you could place it in the category of trust, because your body's feedback is telling you. That said, I would contact customer service and ask them about safety and recommended use during pregnancy. After all of this due diligence, listen to your inner wisdom, and if there is even a whisper of 'no' then don't use it.

Phthalates are used as softeners, or plasticizers, in polyvinyl chloride (PVC, vinyl) products, including children's toys, some teethers, food packaging and cling wrap, medical devices, backpacks, shower curtains, vinyl flooring, wallpaper, decorating and building products, blood bags, adhesives, mosquito insect repellents, plastic plumbing pipes, nail polish, skin moisturizers, perfumes, solvents, cosmetics, personal care products, wood finishes and insecticides. *Studies have found* damaged, shrunken, undescended, or atrophied testicles; reduced sperm production; damaged sperm, destruction of Sertoli cells (which produce sperm) and lowered testosterone levels in offspring where phthalates was present. One great way to avoid Phthalates is to stop drinking water that has been stored in plastic bottles – especially if there is any possibility that it has been exposed to heat.

Arsenic is a naturally occurring element, considered a heavy metal. It is used as a preservative in wood such as pressure-treated lumber for decks, fences, playground equipment and residential construction, in insecticides, weed killers, fungicides, glass production, semiconductors, to make metal alloys (used in lead-acid car batteries), some medications, and home and agricultural fertilizers.

Lead. The most significant sources of lead continue to be from paint in homes built before 1978, lead pipes placed before the 1930s and soil by highways and heavily traveled roads. *Reproductive effects* including decreased fertility, increased rates of miscarriage, pre-term delivery, low birth weight, low sperm count, erectile dysfunction, abnormal sperm shape and size.

Mercury. The most common organic form of mercury in our environment (from volcanoes, coal burning and gold production) accumulates in the flesh of fish, animals and humans, most particularly predatory fish species, such as shark and tuna, and bottom-feeders, such as crab. Animals exposed orally to long-term, high levels of mercury in *laboratory studies* experienced adverse effects on the developing fetus, sperm and male reproductive organs and increases in the number of spontaneous abortions and stillbirths.

24-D is applied to grassy crops such as wheat, lawns and gardens. It can be found on roadsides, golf courses, forests and waterways. If you are a golfer, be sure to bring changes of socks so your feet stay dry and are not sitting in a moist chemical environment for a full 18 holes. Also use a rag to pick up your ball, especially after it has been on the green as this is an area of the course which is most heavily sprayed with chemicals and fertilizers.

Permethrin is an insecticide derived from chrysanthemum flowers. It has multiple uses, including head lice and scabies treatment, insect repellents (including household foggers and sprays), tick and flea sprays for yards and pets, termite treatments, agricultural and livestock products, forestry and timber treatment. There are alternatives that are much less toxic to control these pests, and many insect repellents do not contain this chemical anymore.

Toxic Sludge. This is a term used for the substances that get filtered out of our sewage and water treatment plants. It is comprised of industrial, petro-chemical and pharmaceutical waste as well as heavy metals and plastics. Conventional farmers are now purchasing this Toxic Sludge as fertilizers to spread all over their land in an effort to produce more bountiful harvests. Another fantastic reason to support organic farming, isn't it?

History repeating itself?
Obviously cigarettes, alcohol and drugs are a no-no. When we look to the not-too distant past, smoking in places like maternity wards and airplanes was perfectly acceptable. We may shake our heads in disbelief but I imagine future generations will feel the same way about some of the

things we put in our bodies. From microwaving our food to drinking water from plastic containers and spraying perfume directly on our skin, I'm willing to bet that there will be a level of disbelief at our ignorance from future generations. The best advice really is to do your homework. If your doctor prescribes medication, ask about the side effects and take the initiative to read about them independently. If you see something on a food label and you're not sure what it is, Google it. Knowledge is power!

By creating a clean environment in your own body, you are making it more hospitable for a baby and increasing the health and well-being of your future child. That's worth making some adjustments for, right? It may seem daunting at first, but start small and work your way up. When you have adjusted to changes, choose more to implement. Dedication to your healthier-living path will ensure you are doing your part in protecting your fertility.

Chapter Task:

List three things / products you need to stop using right now:

1. _____

2. _____

3. _____

Write down any questions you still have about toxins in our environment:

_____

_____

_____

_____

Now go and find answers to these questions!

Step Eight

Treatments and Alternatives to Enhance TCM

How to increase your chances of success

"Stay committed to your decisions, but stay flexible in your approach." ~Tony Robbins

---

Here are a few ideas that will compliment Traditional Chinese Medicine and improve your overall health.

Reproductive Clinical Counselling

Trying to conceive and experiencing setbacks brings up a lot of feelings that can be difficult to process independently or even with your partner. Finding someone to talk to that is not directly involved can be very helpful. Reproductive health counselling provides emotional support for all aspects of reproduction from infertility to postpartum depression to recurrent pregnancy loss and IVF support.

An experienced counsellor will give perspective that can be hard to see when you are deeply immersed in the goal of having a child. Find someone with experience and compassion. They will be an invaluable support system.

Q&A with Holly Yager, M.ED. RCC
Well Woman Counselling

Why reproductive health & fertility counselling?

Many of the 1 in 6 Canadian couples who experience infertility consider it to be one of the most stressful times in their lives. In fact, infertility is ranked just as distressing as a diagnosis of a terminal illness, such as cancer (IAAC, 2012). The months (or years) of riding the monthly emotional roller coaster, of coping with treatment failure and pregnancy loss, and of seeing everyone else managing to successfully achieve the dream of raising a family can eventually take its toll.

Infertility can affect mood, stress levels, self-esteem, and overall quality of life. It can bring on spiritual, health, career, financial, and relationship concerns. It is common for couples' relationships to become so focused on fertility that both emotional and sexual intimacy can become compromised. Relationships with others can be affected as well, because many couples keep their fertility struggle to themselves and avoid family gatherings and social events where they may be emotionally triggered. Many women and men who are experiencing infertility report feeling a lack of support from others.

What is reproductive health & fertility counselling?

Reproductive health & fertility counselling addresses the emotional concerns and challenges related to infertility, pregnancy, and hormones. Whether you are trying to conceive, undergoing fertility treatments, coping with miscarriage, or transitioning to pregnancy and parenthood, it is crucial to have support from someone experienced in these matters. A reproductive health & fertility counsellor can provide support and guidance throughout all stages of the reproductive health cycle.

How can reproductive health & fertility counselling help you?

Reproductive health and fertility counselling can help you cope with the stress of infertility, whether trying to conceive naturally or with the use of assisted reproductive technologies (ARTs), such as IVF and IUI. It can also help you while building your family through the use of third-party reproduction, such as donor conception or gestational surrogacy. Reproductive health counselling can help you cope with any fertility-related challenges that may arise, such as maintaining intimacy and communication in relationships, managing stress related to fertility treatments, coping with pregnancy loss, treating anxiety or depression during or after pregnancy, and preparing for childbirth and parenting. If the need arises, a reproductive health counsellor can also provide assistance with the decision to end treatment, to adopt, or to live child-free.

What should you look for in a reproductive health counsellor?

When looking for a professional to help support you during your fertility journey, it is important to make sure that your counsellor is qualified in this area. First, you will want to make sure that your counsellor is graduate-level (Masters or PhD) educated in a mental health discipline from an accredited institution. Your counsellor should also be registered or certified with a professional organization, such as the Canadian Counselling & Psychotherapy Association or the BC Association of Clinical Counsellors. This ensures that your counsellor follows ethical standards of practice and engages in regular professional development. It also ensures that your counsellor uses proven, evidence-based psychotherapies. In addition to providing support, a qualified reproductive health counsellor is trained in the use of psychotherapeutic techniques, such as cognitive behavioural therapy (CBT) or mindfulness-based stress reduction (MBSR).

Acupressure

Another facet of TCM is acupressure. Not unlike acupuncture, acupressure is a tool that is based on the concept that life energy flows through meridians in the body and that by applying pressure at key points, this energy can better flow to clear blockages that may be causing health problems.

My preference is for acupuncture as it offers more in-depth and effective treatment. But for stress, acupressure is ideal in between acupuncture appointments at home or if you live in a rural area where acupuncture isn't available. Acupressure is free and can be done wherever you are once you educate yourself.

Since one of the major factors to less than perfect health is stress, feeling relaxed is paramount to increased fertility. The following are three pressure points that will help with stress and are literally right at your fingertips.

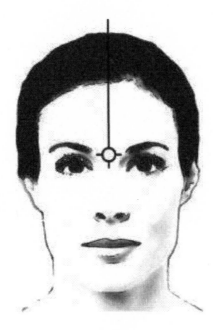

YINTANG

1st point – YINTANG

Sometimes called the "3rd eye" point that is
located on the forehead, dead centre between the
inner edges of both eyebrows. There is usually a
small bone depression at this point, and sometimes
it can feel a bit sensitive. It is easy to know when
you're in the right spot, as the soothing effect is
usually immediate. Wonderful for inducing a
general calm state, it can also help relax a tired
face and eyes, and may help quiet a stress
headache. Adding a gentle circular motion to
pressing this point can increase the effect.

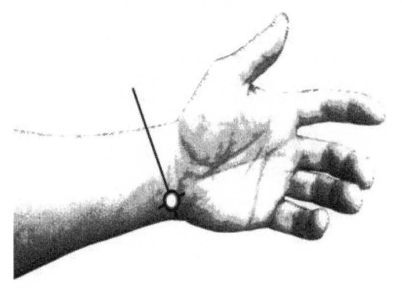

SHENMEN

2nd point – SHENMEN

Also called "Heart 7", this is the source point of the heart, which in Chinese Medicine is thought to govern the mind and spirit. Hold your hand in front of your face with your palm facing you. On your wrist, at the corner of your palm directly below the base of your little finger, you should be able to see or feel a ropey tendon. Place the thumb of your opposite hand on this tendon, and roll your thumb inwards on the wrist. As your thumb sinks into a soft spot, you've found the point. Because it goes to the heart, this point is very useful when stress is causing uncomfortable feelings or palpitations in the chest, and is highly effective in anxiety or panic attacks.

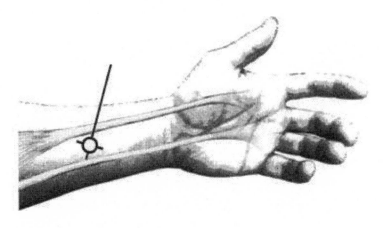

NEIGUAN

3rd point – NEIGUAN

Also called "Pericardium 6", this is a very versatile point that you may recognise from the travel bands people wear for motion sickness. This point is located about 3 finger breadths above the inner crease of the wrist, centred between two major tendons. Not just for motion sickness, this point can be very useful when stress is causing any sort of digestive upset.

Traditional Chinese Medicine holistically restores balance in all systems of the body and when all systems are in a state of balance, fertility potential is realized.

Integrative Life Coaching

An integrative life coach works with individuals and couples to provide solutions and possibilities for achieving a more meaningful life. The goal is to help you move from where you are to where you want to be by helping you realize your strengths and recognizing where you might be self-sabotaging. Sometimes a subtle shift is

179

all someone needs to help them reach their goals and the unbiased opinion of a professional offers insight that you may not otherwise have.

Thomas Dolan, coach on Integrative Coaching:
Unlike traditional counseling or therapy where you look to someone else for guidance, Integrative Coaching guides you to find your own answers. It is a process designed to support becoming whole and expressing oneself. The work opens people up to receiving the wisdom of how they are blocking themselves from claiming the magnificence of creating a life.

Tracy G. on Thomas Dolan:

Working with Thomas has opened up a new world of possibilities and wonder for me. At the heart of our sessions was the connection to my heart center and with this, the actualization of finding my own answers within instead of seeking them from an external source. Initially I was concerned that I wouldn't have any answers, but with gentle coaching and much patience, Thomas supported me time and again in resurrecting latent intuition and hidden gems of insight that could only come from my inner wisdom. Through the work, I have come to greater acceptance of myself, focusing on letting go of societal pressures, owning my power, and uncovering desires or self-expressions that have resulted in a new passion and potential career. All this through taking responsibility for my choices. Life is fuller and more meaningful having worked with Thomas. Thomas has supported my mind, my emotions and my soul with much needed lessons in sticking to facts and releasing my pain-producing stories, along with creating greater peace of mind in the process.

This has been a welcome addition to my fertility treatment focusing on the body with Dr. Spence Pentland, who has also been instrumental in my finding balance physically, holistically and energetically.

See a Chiropractor

A chiropractor will evaluate your physical structure/posture and get you 'straightened out' if need be. When pelvic alignment is off, posture is poor or back issues are apparent, necessary smooth muscle movement of the uterus may be restricted making conception a challenge. It is something that is easy to fix and can be the difference between a baby and no baby, so is definitely worth it!

Dr. Janelle B.
Chiropractor

Susan sits across from me in my office talking excitedly about the weekend ahead, an impromptu trip to the Gulf Islands with her husband. Susan has travelled to almost every continent. She is happily married, loves her job and sports the open, infectious smile of someone who is by all accounts a happy person but this hasn't always been the case. For the first two years of their marriage, Susan and Bryan tried without success to become pregnant naturally. According to Bryan, "It was the hardest thing for us. We always just assumed things would fall into place. It was difficult to go through and left us feeling just so powerless."

Like so many other couples I've seen, the experience lead them to the realization that they might just need a little help. Susan and Bryan are two months into their new plan which includes a modified diet, exercise, IVF, acupuncture and other alternative therapies to put them both in top shape. They've come in to my office on the advice of a friend. Susan's hopes are fragile and delicate after so much disappointment, but she has done some research and would like to know how a chiropractic

181

adjustment could possibly help her get pregnant.

A quick Google search of chiropractic and infertility leads to several case studies and new research on the benefits of chiropractic when trying to resolve fertility issues. Chiropractic is becoming increasingly popular with fertility clinics and couples who are having difficulty conceiving because of the close relationship between the spine and nervous system. When the brain can properly communicate to all organ systems without interference, miracles (or simply, proper function) can happen.

The main reason for a properly functioning reproductive system in both males and females (uterus, fallopian tubes, ovaries, prostate, testicles, etc.) is a good nerve connection from the brain down to all of these different parts. For example, if someone were to cut these nerves, no amount of good nutrition, supplements or even chiropractic adjustments could help these organs heal or even keep them alive. The role of a Chiropractor is to help remove the physical stress on that nerve and restore proper nerve function to the different organ systems.

There are several stressors that can cause interference to messages traveling down to the organs. In my opinion, all should be looked at for overall health and well-being. Whether it's poor nutrition or medications causing chemical stress, tension in the muscles or soft tissue caused by emotional or mental stress, or poor biomechanics of the spine causing physical stress on the nerves, all could be affecting the health of the organs and the entire body.

As a chiropractor, I find and locate the physical stressors coming from a misalignment of the spine or pelvis. Most lower back nerves and sacral nerves innervate the reproductive organs. A full assessment of this area is essential in ensuring a healthy conception and pregnancy.

The entire spine is often looked at as an old injury or current stress in the neck or upper back can also cause interference in the signals traveling down the spine to the reproductive organs.

Susan is like so many women who come in, ready to do everything she can to improve their chances of conceiving. I would love to say that after getting a few simple chiropractic adjustments, conception will happen naturally and easily. No chiropractor can make that prediction, but I can promise that you won't have wasted your time, money or energy. Although I don't know the particular reasons for every instance of infertility, I do know that clearing stress on your central nerve system will help nourish your organs and optimize your overall health, getting your body in the best possible shape to conceive and bringing you one step closer to having a baby. For Susan and her husband, the road to parenthood has been long but they are facing the future more brightly and dreaming that their next big trip will require travel plans for three. I can't wait to get that postcard!

Massage

You will be hard-pressed to find an argument against the stress-relieving qualities of massage. Whether you are experiencing the anxiety of trying to conceive or the changes in your body that pregnancy brings, massage therapy is a highly beneficial indulgence.

It can be used to increase circulation (which is imperative for fertility, particularly in older women), restore a connection to your body, improve posture and prepare you for labour during your pregnancy. All that and it feels fantastic. What's not to love?

Natalie Woodhouse
Registered Massage Therapist

All aspects of a mature adult city life; work, financial, family, relationships, home renovations, school deadlines, health concerns, life changes and other ongoing responsibilities can make the road to pregnancy a stressful one. Clients seeking optimum fertility need to examine how much of their life operates at high stress levels and how much that stress takes away from self-care. This can lead them to tolerating a wide variety of physical discomforts, exhausting the nervous system and disrupting the chemical balance in the body. Common complaints related to chronic tension and stress show up in the neck, head, and shoulders, low back and hip pain, and often in the stomach, or other abdominal or pelvic systems. These complaints are easily aggravated by stress, repetitive daily use, poor posture and lack of activity. Hands-on bodywork ultimately opens our ability for intuitive communication with our body, providing wonderful relief for the nervous system and in turn, hormone management. For people experiencing infertility, the simplicity of a massage therapy treatment can diminish pain and stress levels in the body and mind. This window can significantly relieve stress, anxiety and pain levels long enough for the brain stem and nervous system to do corrective management for hormone regulation.

In one case, a female client came in with physical discomforts in the neck and shoulders, so painful it would often cause nausea. She had been receiving regular acupuncture for fertility but needed further assistance in relieving the muscle spasms. The tension in the neck had been long term, compounded from a series of old car accidents, and most recently aggravated due to the accumulation of stress. The goal of using massage therapy in this case was to help her restore a calm nervous system by resolving the pain and tension in her neck and shoulders so that she could feel a sense of ease and relaxation in her own body. As she settled onto the massage table with deep breathing, the focus was placed on postural alignment to restore to the spine, pelvis and shoulder girdle to help reduce the ongoing heavy ache in her shoulders. Myofascial Release and Neuromuscular therapy were used with a deep tissue Ayurvedic flare to ease painful trigger points in the upper back, neck and sacral area to essentially nurture and soothe the nervous system. Treatments often begin with a basic postural examination to establish the tissue quality in the area of the main complaint and to observe for other whole body factors that could be contributing to the posture dysfunction of the pelvis, spine, cranium and abdominal area. Other Massage techniques that work specifically well for fertility involves working with the abdomen to mobilize the viscera (organs), and the treatments often involve visualization or energy work. The aim of a Yinstill RMT treatment is to balance the nervous system, encourage blood flow, and reducing physical discomforts with hands-on therapy, improving posture to the pelvic organ function.

For those working toward fertility, it would be recommended to receive treatments before, or, after ovulation, or menstruation to help relieve abdominal tension, increase circulation and clear energy blocks held in the body. In this case mentioned above, each individual treatment had a positive relaxing effect on the client but the cumulative effect of the treatments working together is what created the lasting softness to the tissue quality and aided in developing the client's level of body awareness and deeper sense of connection to her posture and self-care. When she returned at a later date, excited about her recent pregnancy, the massage evaluation and techniques were changed again to support her body in nourishing the embryo development. Even without consecutive treatment, the client saw small changes towards correct posture, and had a positive stress-free experience, contributing to her ultimate goal of pregnancy.

If you're undergoing expensive infertility treatments, spending money on anything that doesn't directly involve eggs and sperm may seem unnecessary and excessive, but consider the amount of stress and tension your body is going through and give yourself permission to get an occasional massage. The relaxation will do your body good. Developing a health care plan that includes massage and other body therapies is important to help maintain quality of life and encourages healthy function of major systems like fertility.

Top three things to consider in how massage can benefit fertility:

1. *A harmonious sonata happens between your nerves and hormones as you relax into your massage. A gentle shift in stimulation of the nervous system from 'fight or flight' to 'rest and digest' can change the function that nurtures the activities of hormones that play a big role in fertility success.*

2. *Abdominal massage and deep breathing can act as a pump for the lymphatic system and blood flow in the lower abdomen allowing for delivery of essential nutrients to developing follicles and supporting organs.*

3. *The benefits of structural support and postural adjustments will result in pain relief and less stress on muscles and bones that may have been compensating.*

Massage for Common Pregnancy Aches & Pains

Once you get pregnant (and I have faith you will), your body will be undergoing some major changes as everything inside of you shifts to make room for baby--and that's just the physical aspect. Additionally, nervousness and stress are not uncommon as your life is about to undergo a complete transformation but prolonged or severe stress can cause complications, so self-care is of utmost importance during this time. Make time to rest, breathe deeply and get massages. Learn to love your special moments of peace and relaxation as you receive treatment.

Utilize massage during pregnancy for relief of many common aches and pains. Here is just a just a few examples of what we see on the massage table seeking relief:

- *Lower back and hip ache*
- *Upper back and neck ache*
- *Pain under the ribs*
- *Pubic pain*
- *Pain in the groin*
- *Numbness and tingling in the hands*
- *Recurring night cramps in the legs*

Visiting your massage therapist regularly, every two to four weeks, will make a big difference in your overall well-being after baby arrives too. You will be doing a lot of giving to your newborn, and taking some time to give to yourself should not be forgotten.

Increasing Blood Flow to the Reproductive Organs

Optimal circulation to the reproductive organs is essential for men and women to maximize fertility and decrease miscarriage since blood delivers nutrition and oxygen where needed.

Sluggish blood flow can be caused by stress, a lack of exercise, not enough rest or joy and even certain foods. All the usual culprits! Here are a few ways to turn it around.

Castor Oil Packs

A castor oil pack can be placed on the skin to increase circulation and promote elimination and healing of the tissues and organs; in this case, the ovaries and uterus. I recommend doing it in the evenings with a hot water foot soak as outlined below. It is a great way to have some relaxation time that is also productive.

The best timing for this is during the ten days of the follicular phase of your menstrual cycle (approximately days 3 through 12).

The packs are made by soaking a small piece of flannel or cotton about the size of a folded facecloth in castor oil and placing it on the skin immediately above the pubic hair line. A hot water bottle is then placed on top of the cloth for 30-60 minutes to heat the oil, aiding in absorption.

Be sure and rest while the pack is in place. After removal, cleanse your stomach with a diluted solution of water and baking soda. Store the cloth in a covered container in the refrigerator. There is no need to wash it; the oil can be left on for its next use.

NOTE: *Castor oil should not be taken internally. It should not be applied to broken skin or used* *during pregnancy and breastfeeding.*

Hot Water Foot Soak

Great to do in concert with castor oil packs as an evening ritual. Research shows that hot water foot baths at 49 degrees Celsius (120 degrees Fahrenheit) can be very beneficial to a woman's fertility by increasing blood flow to the reproductive organs. Every night before bed, especially during the follicular phase (i.e., approximately days 3 through 12) of the menstrual cycle, give your feet some love! Run your hot water tap for one minute. Most water furnaces are set to approximately 120-140 degrees but if it feels far too hot, check the temperature. Fill a container large enough to fit both feet, then kick back and relax for 15-20 minutes.

Femoral massage

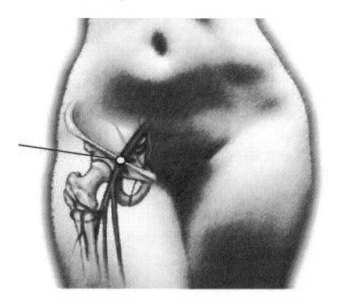

This is a great way to provide nourishment to the

Dr. Spence Pentland

uterus, ovaries, testes and penis. You can do this massage on your own (but having a partner perform is best) by following these few simple steps.

The femoral artery is located level with your pubic bone, just beneath the crease in your groin between your thigh and lower abdomen.

To begin, compress the femoral artery with your fingers using fairly heavy pressure. When you feel the flow has ceased, hold for 30 seconds. The blood will then back up and increase the pressure gradient in the iliac arteries which forces more blood into the pelvic arteries. This floods the pelvic organs and genitals with more blood. When the hold is released, you should feel a sensation of warmth rushing down your legs as the blood supply returns to the lower extremities.

Women should perform femoral massage from the end of menses to ovulation or retrieval date if undergoing IVF. Do 2-3 times each leg, 1-2 times per day. It is actually even better if the woman can relax while their partner does the massage.

CAUTION: Do not perform this exercise if you are pregnant, are post-transfer during an IVF cycle, have high blood pressure, have heart disease or circulatory problems such as aneurysms, varicose veins, phlebitis or thrombosis, have a history of strokes or detached retinas.

Get Happy!

I've talked about stress and its unkind cousins like anxiety and hopelessness in Step Four, but it cannot be overstated that finding happiness will make all the difference in the world to your fertility.

Books on Happiness

- ♥ *The Happiness Project by Gretchen Rubin*
- ♥ *Bright Side Up: 100 Ways to be Happier Right Now by Amy Spencer*
- ♥ *Stumbling on Happiness by Daniel Gilbert*

Nine times out of ten, unexplained fertility is found to be emotional so let go of stress and find what makes you happy instead. Not that there is anything wrong with feeling a range of feelings. Having difficulty starting a family is bound to bring up lots of emotions, but be mindful of how you deal with them. When you feel your frustration rising, make a conscious effort to talk to someone supportive or take a bike ride or whatever it is that makes you feel better. Bottling things up will eat away at you and your chances of conception.

Story
Amberlie K.

The miscarriage and 2nd failed IVF really changed me. I'm not sure if it was harder than the first time in that I actually had so much hope the 2nd time around. I felt like I climbed to a cliff and then fell off. For months, I just felt like I was falling. The pain was so great I couldn't put words to it. Not even to myself. I'd experienced depression before but it had never "broken my brain" as it did this time. I couldn't remember things, was confused constantly, didn't sleep and felt no connection to anything important in my life. I managed to form feelings in pictures rather than words, which became many drawings where houses or trees were floating in space - no ground beneath them. Another recurrent image was of me with my

191

mouth full of rocks. In many ways I still feel like my mouth is full of rocks. It is so hard to talk about what happened, how I feel, what it means for my future...

I have been going to see a wonderful counselor and she has helped a lot. I also have many loving people around me who have cared for me in this vulnerable time. I know I'm not alone, and that helps. Slowly, I have found a measure of healing. I'm still learning to care and extend the grace for myself in the way I do for others. I've found joy and connection in my life again.

I think about being a mother still. How can I not? But I approach those thoughts with incredible caution. We have 4 embryos left, which would be 2 attempts at conception. I'm still too terrified to return to PCRM. I've just recently found the ground under my feet. I don't want to lose it again.

My counselor said to me recently that perhaps I don't need to "feel" a certain way to go through the procedures with the embryos, instead I can just see them as doors to go through to lead through to the next step. If we conceive, that would be a miracle. If we don't, we would be choosing to move on to adoption. It feels like a bit of a relief to not hinge so much emotion on the procedures, but it's a hard thing to do for a person who is an innate 'feeler'. Obviously, I need to feel healthy, positive and whole when I do pursue those procedures, so this is what I'm working on day by day. Taking care of me. Finding value in who I am by what I have, rather than what I don't have.

Chapter Task:

Decide on one new Complementary/Alternative Medicine treatment you will try this week:

1. _____

Write down any questions you have about these other treatment types:

_____

_____

_____

_____

Now go and find answers to these questions!

Step Nine

Assisted Reproductive Technology (ART):

The ins and outs of integrating TCM with IVF

"Miracles come in moments. Be ready and willing."
~Wayne Dyer

W omen and couples come to me at various stages of their journey to conception. Sometimes they have been trying for years and others they are just starting out. While conceiving naturally is everyone's first choice, alternatives that garner the same results, a baby, should not be overlooked. It is for this reason that I have included this chapter.

Assisted Reproductive Technology (ART) is a term used to describe the current western medical treatments available for women and couples having difficulty conceiving and desiring or requiring medical aid such as In Vitro Fertilization (IVF).

With current changes in cultural perceptions regarding IVF, and consistent advancement including better freezing techniques, better embryo culture, ways to choose embryos, pre-implantation genetic diagnosis (PGD) and new drugs, IVF is becoming more and more common. I am happy to work with women that choose this route and to implement treatment that aids in their success.

Forward thinking IVF clinics are forming strong alliances with TCM practitioners (with the integration of procedures such as acupuncture). They realize that in addition to successful IVF outcomes, traditional practices enhance the patient's experience by managing stress and cultivating emotional balance.

I am inspired by the integration and kinship that has grown between my practice and that of the local IVF clinics and I am glad to hear of similar relationships being formed elsewhere. We all share the goal of building happy families and by working together, the patient is looked at as a whole and better supported along their journey. This is the growth of great medicine.

A recent article by Michael Fiorani and Dr. Paul Magarelli reviewed the mechanisms and published clinical trials supporting the use of acupuncture with ART and determined that acupuncture should be considered as a viable adjunct therapy for IVF. Their conclusion states:

> *"The use of acupuncture for infertility as an adjunct therapy to conventional treatment in ART (mainly as an adjunct to IVF) has continued to increase in popularity through evidence-based publications demonstrating clinical efficacy. Although acupuncture is based on ancient medical theory, an increasing number of published scientific studies show that acupuncture positively impacts fertility and IVF success rates due to possible mechanisms influencing the menstrual cycle through B-endorphin secretion, affecting gonadotropin secretion through their action on GnRH. These possible mechanisms also impact uterine and ovarian blood flow, cytokines and depression, anxiety and stress. Retrospective and randomized controlled trials have found that acupuncture has a statistically significant positive*

*impact on IVF success rates, including
implantation, pregnancy, and live birth rates,
while reducing the number of miscarriages and
ectopic pregnancies."*

The article also clearly summarized possible mechanisms
of how acupuncture positively impacts fertility and IVF
success rates:

1. *Affects the hypothalamus-pituitary-ovarian
    hormonal axis causing changes in the
    menstrual cycle (through the secretion of b-
    endorphins which affect gonadotropin-
    releasing hormone [GnRH])*
2. *Improving uterine and ovarian blood flow*
3. *Secreting cytokines and regulating the immune
    system*
4. *Relief of depression, anxiety and stress*

Supporting ART treatments with TCM is advantageous in
many ways for the patient. Below is evidence (made up of
over 5000 women in various trials) that shows how
acupuncture administered on the day of embryo transfer
immediately before and after the procedure can
significantly improve success rates.

- Oxford Journals Human Reproduction:
  *Acupuncture administered on the day of embryo
  transfer is most advantageous for those patients
  whose chance of success with IVF is not high*
  (Manheimer, 2013).
- Fertility and Sterility: *Acupuncture improves
  clinical pregnancy rates and live birth rates
  among women undergoing IVF. Increased positive
  effects from using acupuncture in IVF can be
  expected if more reasonable acupuncture
  programs are used* (Zheng, 2012).
- Cochrane Database of Systematic Reviews:
  Acupuncture on the day of Embryo Transfer

improves the ongoing pregnancy rate and the clinical pregnancy rate (Cheong, 2008).

- British Medical Journal: *Current preliminary evidence suggests that acupuncture increased the odds of clinical pregnancy by 65%, and improved live birth rates when compared with the control groups* (Manhheimer, 2008).

Time permitting, researchers Magarelli/Cridennda found that it is optimal to work with TCM for a period of at least 9 consecutive acupuncture treatments before embarking on western medical reproductive treatments. The appropriate time frame for pre-IVF/TCM care depends on the pre-existing conditions the woman or couple has. By helping women regulate their menstrual cycle, lose weight, reduce stress, regulate hormones (Zhou 2013, Magarelli/Cridennda 2009) and increase blood flow (nutrition, oxygen, and medications) to the ovaries, eggs, and uterine lining (Stener-Victorin, 1996 & 2003), TCM plays an important role in the optimization of overall reproductive health and well-being.

Acupuncture and IVF Patients

"Acupuncture could benefit IVF patients beyond potentially improving rates of IVF pregnancy success, noting that it is safe and inexpensive and may aid these patients in coping with the emotional and psychological challenges related to IVF and fertility."
- Excerpted from the Oxford Journals Human Reproduction Meta-analysis by Manheimer et al, 2013.

An assessment of patient demand and importance of acupuncture to patients of an IVF fertility clinic in the UK during lead up, procedures and treatment published in 'Human Fertility' surveyed 200 patients (*Hinks, 2010*).

They discovered that there was a clear demand for acupuncture and that this treatment may be valuable in improving the general well-being of women during infertility and IVF lead up, procedures and treatment. They also felt that patient resilience may be increased by the use of acupuncture when used in conjunction with their IVF treatment such that patients would persevere with increased numbers of IVF cycles, thereby increasing their ultimate chance of starting or expanding their family.

Patience

IVF is a groundbreaking treatment. It helps get women pregnant that may never have been able to do so otherwise. It is truly a miracle of modern science that fulfills the dreams of so many women and couples, but if you are young and healthy and if your fertility specialist recommends continuing to try to conceive naturally, should you choose IVF to hasten the process, or give TCM a chance.?

If you can find the patience to utilize TCM to prepare your body for the journey of pregnancy before resorting to IVF, you may be pleasantly surprised that you become pregnant naturally. And if not, you have optimized your body mind and spirit for success with your IVF.

Being impatient, according to Traditional Chinese Medicine, is a major cause of infertility struggles and is often a key trait of the women that are diagnosed with 'unexplained infertility'. This is a symptom that responds very favorably to TCM and is of primary importance to balance with our treatment. Your child will come when she or he is ready; have faith.

After speaking with Julie Indichova (author of 'Inconceivable') and listening to her speak, she inspired the following important message: *Before stepping into*

IVF, please be ready on all levels; become one with your body mind and spirit. If you haven't already done so, stop seeing conception or your body as something that needs to be accomplished or conquered. Have faith that your body knows how and that your baby will come. Be as loving to yourself as you would be to your child. This may be difficult, but it is an appropriately tailored assignment when planning for IVF success.

Conceiving Naturally After IVF

"Be thankful for what you have; you'll end up having more." ~Oprah Winfrey

Some interesting studies:

- One in three women who have their first baby through infertility treatment become pregnant again naturally within two years of their first birth (Wynter, 2013).

- A Monash University study, published in the Australian and New Zealand Journal of Obstetrics and Gynecology, was the first to examine the rates of unexpected conception in Australian women who had a first child through assisted reproductive technology such as IVF. The study of 236 women who had a baby through assisted reproductive treatments found 33 percent of them conceived a second child naturally within two years of their first birth and women whose infertility was initially diagnosed as 'unexplained' were more than twice as likely as others with a specific infertility diagnosis to become pregnant naturally.

To me, these findings make perfect sense, especially unexplained infertility, which 9 times out of 10 in traditional Chinese medicine carries a huge emotional component. Once a woman has started her family, the pressure lifts and baby number two often comes easily. Deep internal blockage is removed and life flows a little more smoothly. According to Traditional Chinese Medicine, we call it coursing the liver and rectifying the qi.

If you have been trying for some time for your first child and are considering IVF, I suggest taking some time to prepare with TCM. Nourish the soil before planting the seed. From my experience, this can sometimes make IVF unnecessary.

Adhering to the recommendations of this book may not only help you conceive, but will create a healthy environment for your future child. By improving your diet, minding your stress and getting proper exercise and fulfillment, you will be optimizing your chances of of a healthy and happy family, be it naturally or with ART.

The Ideal Time for TCM if Considering IVF

- If you are overweight: The importance of a healthy BMI before attempting an IVF cannot be overstated. Take the time and make a commitment. Use the vision of your dream family to cultivate a compelling reason to dedicate to stepping up. Make it the first great parenting decision you make and the first example you set for your children.
- Unexplained Infertility: This can be a frustrating diagnosis and most often involves a large degree of emotional stagnation and stress. In my experience, this is far more common in couples in their early 30's. Acupuncture administered consistently for 4-12 weeks before the IVF embryo transfer has proven to be very beneficial.
- Recurrent Pregnancy Loss: If you are getting pregnant easily but miscarrying, TCM is a good

option to utilize in an attempt to correct the issues that may be contributing to the recurrent loss. A study of 238 women undergoing IVF treatment showed those who received acupuncture had significantly less first trimester miscarriages when compared to the women that did not receive acupuncture (*Khorram et al 2012*). IVF itself does not help reduce miscarriage unless pre-implantation genetic diagnosis (PGD) is implemented.

- Stress: Our preliminary clinical data tells us that acupuncture administered consistently, 4-12 weeks before the IVF embryo transfer, significantly reduces stress levels.
- Thin uterine lining: Evidence based research demonstrates that acupuncture, done correctly, increases blood flow to the reproductive organs such as uterus and ovaries (as noted in studies by Stener-Victorin in 1996 & 2003). I have seen problematic thin uterine linings that would potentially delay or cancel many IVF cycles thicken significantly with just a few acupuncture treatments.

Basic TCM Treatment Recommendations:
- In most cases, 13-14 acupuncture treatments in the 2.5-3 months prior to embryo transfer is ideal. This recommendation is based on our own clinical data and experience cross referenced with current peer recommendations and available research cited throughout this chapter. This can vary depending on pre-existing conditions. It may be extremely beneficial if appropriate and time permits to give up to six months or more before an IVF cycle when a woman needs to lose weight or has multiple hormonal imbalances and irregular menstrual cycles such as with PCOS.
- Two acupuncture treatments per week during

stimulation injections. This is a time to work on three main things: 1. increasing medication delivery to the ovaries, 2. improving the quality and thickness of the uterine lining, and 3. managing stress.

- On site (at IVF clinic) acupuncture immediately before and after embryo transfer. A number of studies cited earlier (Manheimer 2008 & 2013, Zheng 2012, Cheong 2008) which displayed improved pregnancy and live birth rates involved the administration of acupuncture immediately before then again immediately after the embryo transfer on site at the IVF clinic. I will touch on the importance of on-site embryo transfer day acupuncture more below.

- Acupuncture once per week throughout the first trimester of pregnancy. Supportive treatments, particularly during the emotional two-week waiting period post embryo transfer when a woman has to go home and patiently await the arrival of her pregnancy test results or her menses. Then throughout pregnancy as continued emotional support (especially for those who have suffered recurrent loss) and for conditions along the way such as nausea, aches and pains, high blood pressure and in the unfortunate case of miscarriage. Finally, preparation for labour and delivery from week 36 onward is highly recommended.

Options for ART

In Vitro Fertilization (IVF) is a method of assisted reproduction that involves a protocol of drugs and injectable hormones to stimulate the growth of ovarian follicles that contain the eggs and then combines the eggs retrieved from the ovaries with sperm in a laboratory dish. If the eggs fertilize and cell division progresses properly, the healthiest looking embryos are transferred into the woman's uterus where they will hopefully implant in the uterine lining and further develop into a baby. IVF bypasses the fallopian tubes and is usually the treatment choice for women who have badly damaged or absent tubes. However, in recent years, IVF has become a popular option for whomever desires to utilize this technology.

ICSI (Intracytoplasmic sperm injection) is an advanced form of IVF most often used when sperm quality is poor. It is a process like IVF with the exception of how the eggs are fertilized. In IVF, the eggs and sperm are put together in a petri dish and allowed to court one another, almost the same way it would happen in the fallopian tube. In ICSI, an embryologist chooses sperm with a microscopic syringe and manually injects it into the egg (fertilization).

IUI (Intra Uterine Insemination) is a relatively simple process compared to others that involves the collection and injection of sperm into the uterus. It is a technique used with or without the aid of medications to stimulate the ovaries to produce more eggs. In many respects, this is a first step into ART, or simply the path to pregnancy if using donor sperm.

Clomid (clomiphene citrate or similar medications such as Letrozole - trade name 'Femara') are drugs taken orally for five days near the beginning of a menstrual cycle that tell the brain to send out more messenger hormones to the ovaries, making them produce more mature eggs helping to induce ovulation. This is the first step in ART fertility treatments as family doctors and gynecologists are allowed to prescribe this class of medication. These drugs are most often used in women with irregular cycles due to conditions like PCOS. They tend to have the secondary effect of supporting the luteal phase (second half of the menstrual cycle) by helping the body produce more mature eggs thus leaving behind a stronger corpus luteum resulting in higher progesterone levels. Clomid may be beneficial for women who have been diagnosed with a luteal phase defect or are not ovulating.

FET (Frozen Embryo Transfers) are frozen embryos from a previous IVF or ICSI cycle that are transferred into the uterus post thaw. Currently, because of its improved technology and success rates, embryo vitrification is being used (instead of traditional freezing methods) as a preservation technique similar to that of freezing. Embryos are also only being frozen if they are of sufficient quality to live to Day 5 or 6 post-egg retrieval. Some IVF clinics prefer this technique over fresh IVF embryo transfers for various reasons, such as ovarian hyperstimulation or the possible benefits of giving the body and mind a break between medications and procedures and the actual transfer of the embryos believing it may provide for a more healthy environment conducive to pregnancy. This can also be used for banking cycles and when a woman wants to use preimplantation genetic diagnostics.

Donor Egg Cycles are a final step in Assisted Reproductive Technologies. They are recommended when a doctor believes a woman will not be able to achieve pregnancy using her own eggs. If a couple feels they can afford this option (which often runs upward of $30,000) it almost promises a baby. The couple finds a woman who will donate her eggs to be fertilized in vitro with the husband's sperm. The resulting embryos are transferred into a healthy and thick estrogen-prepared uterine lining of the mother-to-be. The laws and cost of donor cycles are very different in the USA and Canada and should be researched thoroughly.

A woman emailed me regarding what she was interpreting as a poor response to her IVF cycle. The following was my response. It sums up the trend I see happening with some progressive fertility specialists I know:

High numbers of eggs are not necessarily what we want to be striving for, Jane. Often when numbers are the goal, we end up seeing many immature eggs that don't fertilize or don't grow far enough for transfer. When less eggs are stimulated, your body is reacting more naturally, therefore we can have faith that these should be more quality eggs resulting in similar or better chances of success (i.e., a baby) than if you were to stimulate more eggs. Do not be discouraged and press on to have them transfer. Stay positive and confident. Many fertility doctors I know would be happy with your progress so far.

Preimplantation Genetic Diagnosis (PGD) or Comprehensive Chromosomal Screening (CCS) & Banking Cycles. Due to its impressive improvement of pregnancy rates and reduction of miscarriage rates in high risk women, PGD is gaining popularity. Preimplantation genetic diagnosis (PGD) refers to genetic profiling of embryos prior to implantation. PGD is an adjunct to assisted reproductive technology, and requires in vitro fertilization (IVF) to obtain embryos for evaluation. The two main purposes for use are: 1. determine genetically normal embryos for transfer during an IVF cycle, and 2. to screen for disease or other abnormalities.

I recently went to a talk given by Santiago Munne of

Reprogenetics in New York. He is a pioneer in the development and research of PGD. He clearly demonstrated how this new technology can help improve the success of the current available technologies used in assisted reproduction. For some, it may be cost prohibitive as it adds approximately $5000 to the IVF cycle, but for those that can afford it, especially those who suffer from recurrent pregnancy loss, this may be a very good option. For women that have diminished ovarian reserve, meaning that they will not produce many eggs when stimulated by IVF medications, 'banking' is being recommended more and more, especially if PDG is being considered. Banking means going through multiple IVF cycles but instead of transferring embryos 3 to 5 days after retrieval, they are vitrified (frozen) and this same process is done again and again until there are enough viable embryos making it worthwhile to have them put through comprehensive chromosomal screening (PGD) to find the 'normal' ones to use in a future transfer. Though costly, it is comparable in price to a donor egg cycle.

Frequently Asked Questions

What are the recommendations for acupuncture treatment during an IVF cycle?

- 1 acupuncture treatment per week in the weeks/months leading up to the IVF cycle for both men and women. 9-14 treatments in the 6-12 weeks prior to IVF improves chances of positive outcomes.
- 2 acupuncture treatments per week while undergoing IVF stimulation injection for both men and women.
- On site acupuncture treatments (at IVF clinic) immediately before and after embryo transfer (see below).
- Continued acupuncture 1 per week throughout the

first trimester of pregnancy.

How does acupuncture help with an IVF cycle?

- Improves blood flow to ovaries and uterine lining (delivering nutrition, oxygen, and necessary medications used for various A.R.T. protocols).
- Reduces stress and improves overall experience of the IVF treatment.
- Helps correct imbalances in health that may be inhibiting conception.

Why is it good to have acupuncture between retrieval and transfer?

- Reduces inflammation and bloating caused by the retrieval procedure.
- Increases blood flow to uterine lining and aids in healing.
- Relieves stress and soothes emotions.

How does acupuncture help 3-7 days post embryo transfer?

- Reduces stress and soothes emotions.
- Gently increases blood flow to uterus and embryo (delivering nutrition, oxygen, and necessary medications).
- Creates an environment favorable to implantation.

Why do you do on site acupuncture treatment (on embryo transfer day) instead of at your personal clinic?

- Read on...

On-site Embryo Transfer Day Acupuncture: The Importance of Treatment at the IVF Clinic

Several studies cited earlier have shown that pregnancy rates improve when acupuncture is done the same day an embryo is transferred, with an acupuncture treatment just before the procedure and again afterward.

In all but one of these studies, the acupuncture was administered on site at the IVF clinic.

In the case of the study where the acupuncture that was administered off site (Craig, 2007), in contrast to previous reports, acupuncture before and after embryo transfer was associated with lower biochemical and clinical pregnancy rates when compared to the control group. This outcome was hypothesized to have occurred due to the increased stress associated with navigating busy traffic and a more tightly-packed schedule, when ideally before and after embryo transfer should be a time of rest and relaxation.

Embryo transfer day is potentially very stressful as a lot of factors culminate to hopefully achieve the ultimate goal of pregnancy. Whatever can be done to alleviate stress and improve the chances of success should absolutely be done.

While acupuncture is tremendous for helping hopeful parents to relax, the weeks leading up to the embryo transfer day cannot be overlooked. In my experience, they actually have more impact on positive outcomes and stress levels than does acupuncture the day of transfer. The acupuncture is only one part of an individualized program to properly prepare both the man and the woman for their IVF cycle.

According to the results of our recent clinical research (retrospective cohort) using the Perceived Stress Scale developed by Sheldon Cohen that can be viewed at http://en.wikipedia.org/wiki/Perceived_Stress_Scale, women who are treated with acupuncture at our clinic for >1 month prior to their IVF embryo transfer experience significantly lower stress levels than women who get > 1 month of acupuncture treatments at other non-reproductive focused clinics or women who opted for acupuncture treatments on embryo transfer day only (using a p < 0.05 as a measure of significance). These findings, when cross-referenced with a study done at Stanford (Turner, 2013) that used the same Perceived Stress Scale which concluded: *"Women with lower stress and anxiety levels on the day prior to egg retrieval had a higher pregnancy rate. These results emphasize the need to investigate stress reduction modalities throughout the IVF cycle."*

This clearly displays the important role acupuncture can play in optimizing chances of IVF success.

Laser vs. Needle Acupuncture for Embryo Transfer

We sometimes get asked whether we use laser acupuncture to support clients on embryo transfer day, and the answer is no. At the time of this publication, approximately 20 quality studies (as summarized in the systematic reviews cited earlier) have been done regarding the administration of traditional needle acupuncture on embryo transfer day during an IVF cycle.

From this list, there has only been one study (Fratterelli, 2008) that included the use of laser acupuncture. This particular study reported an increase in implantation rates with the use of laser acupuncture, however, the data also showed little difference in 'ongoing pregnancy rates' between traditional manual needle acupuncture and laser acupuncture. Therefore, until much more research is done and displays further benefit, and most importantly, no harm from laser acupuncture, we choose to administer the evidence supported technique of traditional manual needle acupuncture for all on site embryo transfer day acupuncture treatments.

What people are saying:

"I was thankful for the treatment before and after the transfer. Because it was onsite, it was only a few feet away, which meant more time to let the embryo "snuggle in". It greatly helped to relieve all the tension that I felt leading up to the transfer."

"Having the clinic onsite is great, helps decrease some of the stress of having to drive around to places and make it for the transfer on time. Loved it ! Having Dr. Pentland there was calming for me because he'd been there right from the beginning with us. I went into the transfer very relaxed and I'm certain it contributed to our success."

"The acupuncture was helpful in that it was relaxing and it took my mind off the transfer. The heated bed and blanket was quite nice as the room is somewhat cool. I felt well taken care of."

"I found the whole experience to be very relaxing. I would highly recommend listening to the IVF meditation mp3 that Dr. Pentland suggested before embryo transfer. It made what could have been a stressful day a very positive experience. I was also very appreciative that he was on site and that there was such a smooth transition to the embryo transfer procedure."

"After 6 rounds of Clomid and a failed IVF cycle, I explored the option of IVF acupuncture for my second IVF cycle. Having acupuncture on my embryo transfer day gave me the confidence that my body and mind were at their epitome of relaxation. Also, having it done on site gave me the calming, positive and warm thoughts I was

seeking for the moments leading up to my embryo transfer - and the relaxation right after. I am currently 22 weeks pregnant with twins. I truly believe Dr. Pentland's help has contributed to my success!"

Story
Jilly T.

My husband and I married late, so I was 38 when we started trying to conceive. Having had a sister who had some challenges getting pregnant, I was very aware of the fact that it might not "just happen". After six months with no result, I thought that alternative medicine might be a way to improve our chances.

TCM was my first step. I was intending to also pursue some form of western fertility treatment, but was unsure of what the protocol was going to be. Yinstill came to me as a recommendation and it was my first exposure to Chinese Medicine. Spence helped me to approach my efforts from a wholistic perspective, and gave me the feeling that I was doing things that would improve my ability to get pregnant. I had a few basic things to work on such as weight loss, cleansing and adding dietary supplements.

We also implemented weekly acupuncture sessions when we discussed and worked on the emotional side to the approach. Helping me to reduce stress and get myself in the right mindset was a big part of our work together. I was at the clinic once a week, and during these sessions, Spence and I would usually spend around half an hour breaking down any challenges I'd had that week or he would answer the onslaught of questions I came with, which I was always grateful for.

I got rid of a lot of unhealthy behaviors like junk food, eating late, sleeping too little, drinking and high caffeine

213

intake. I infused a lot of healthy behaviors too. I went to bed early, drank more water, exercised on a daily basis and meditated. I also walked a lot more as a form of de-stressing and I found myself being more present and acquired an inner calm. My energy levels were higher and I generally became a much healthier lady.

One of the aspects of this treatment that I think is so valuable is the attention to attitude. After having watched friends work through the challenges of infertility, I look at Yinstill as my secret (or not so secret as I tell anyone who will listen) weapon as to why I had success on the first try with IVF. I value very highly the importance of a positive attitude in life and am sure that it was instrumental in my success. I think it's a basic tenet of TCM but so often overlooked in western medicine, which is too bad because I know that a lot of women trying to get pregnant would benefit from the advice and attitude adjustment.

I'm usually pretty good at rolling with the punches, and have always been pretty thankful for the life I've had; warts and all. I decided a long time ago that life unfolds as it should and that if mine didn't have kids in it because of the decisions I'd made, it had to be okay. To me, children weren't an absolute unless I had the right partner to have them with, but of course, when the reality of that possibly appears, it's a lot harder to accept. I'd found the right partner, but was 39 and knew the odds might be against me.

Before the treatment, I think my anxiety about being able to conceive was pretty deep in my subconscious. It was there though and reared its head during my consultations for sure. I looked forward to tears during counseling sessions as they let me release any anxiety or doubt. But being a primary teacher and someone that loves kids, I didn't see other children and burst into tears or anything. I just knew I wanted it for myself and it was the first time that potentially even if I did everything I could to make it happen, it still might not.

Fortunately though, I was able to safely carry twins to term, one boy and one girl. They are currently 6 months old and keeping me and my husband pretty busy. I think our relationship was strengthened by the struggle. Being older when we met, we both went into it knowing that children weren't a definite for us, but that we both wanted to have kids. The financial strain is always hard for couples, but I don't think it affected our relationship in any way. My husband was very supportive of the work I did to improve my health for fertility's sake. I often overhear him telling other people about how much I did to make it happen, and he also believes that's what really made our pregnancy happen and what a wonderful moment to see TWO little squishy embryos at the 7 week ultrasound!

We don't plan on having any more children as the hands are pretty full right now, and we feel very blessed. Having babies is challenging, and the shift into your identity as a mother isn't as instantaneous as I'd thought it would be. I didn't really know who I was anymore, and it was weird to be flung into this life that I'd wanted so badly, only to feel completely overwhelmed and wondering if I had made a huge mistake. For me, the first few months was really about basic survival, for Mommy and babies! I didn't feel like I had that time to really bond with them and connect. At some point though, your confidence grows or maybe you just get to know each other, and then all of a sudden the lingering looks at each other, the gentle hand stroking your face, the love in your child's eyes lets you know it's all been worth it and always will be.

You just see love.

Story
Mandeep K

My husband, Dan and I started trying to have a baby when I was 29 years old in 2007. We were pretty relaxed about it and didn't ever suspect that there would be a speed bump in trying to conceive. Actually, I always thought that I was very fertile given my family history and that I would get pregnant immediately after coming off my birth control pills but after 9 months of trying, I had a funny feeling that something just wasn't right. Despite my hormonal blood work and a perfect menstruation cycle, we were not getting pregnant. My family doctor also checked my husband and between the both of us, everything seemed to be normal.

My family doctor referred us to a fertility clinic in October 2008 to re-evaluate and make sure everything was still okay. After all kinds of tests and being scoped and poked, everything seemed to check out. I was repeatedly reminded that I was 30 years old--very young still and should not worry. We started off with IUI and Clomid in October 2008, then again in November with a final try in January of 2009. All three did not work out. I was still trying to be open-minded and ok with the results but I was disappointed. I kept a positive outlook and kept moving forward.

In March 2009 we tried our first IVF. I was put on a drug protocol that was appropriate for my age. It was very challenging and I was nervous, but I was excited because I thought that this was it--I was finally going to be pregnant. Both of us being pharmacists, we were very optimistic because we were taking a medical approach and using a definite science. I was convinced that IVF was going to work!

After all the needles, injections and ultrasounds, we

finally were ready for egg retrieval. I produced 9 eggs. I had no idea what to expect and I thought 9 was good. The next morning I was waiting for the phone call from the lab to tell me how my little embryos were doing. The embryologist said, "I'm sorry, you have no embryos. All the eggs retrieved were fragmented and were very poor quality. But there is one premature egg that we will try to inject using ICSI." I was shocked. I didn't know what to say. I was not expecting this at all. The next morning they called us in to have the 4-cell embryo transferred using the premature egg. I tried to remain optimistic, but it didn't work.

Our follow-up appointment resulted in a diagnosis: poor egg quality – unknown cause due to genetic or environmental factors. WTF! I was not ready for that. The doctor told us to try again and perhaps changing the medication protocol may help the outcome and for MY AGE, I should have produced more than a dozen eggs, not just 9. I was very angry and upset. I was put on a drug protocol which would be for a women in her 40's. The doctor also had suggested to try donor eggs and I absolutely lost it! I would need years of counseling to accept that I would not have my own DNA in this child. I will never forget that conversation.

Since it was so intense, we decided to wait for 3 months to try IVF again. This decision came about after we saw an advertisement in the Genesis clinic's waiting room for fertility acupuncture. We asked the doctor and he said that we could try it but not to fully rely on acupuncture to become pregnant. We attended an information session and started TCM. My time at the clinic was very relaxing and I felt that the treatments were helping me at a different medical level. The little issues I had hormonally (feeling cold all the time, light periods, severe cramping, etc.) were slowly being resolved. I decided to do weekly acupuncture sessions. During the entire fertility journey I continued acupuncture weekly, primarily with Dr. Erin Flynn over the years and also numerous times with Spence as well. Both great clinicians.

Then, in September 2009 I became pregnant – NATURALLY! While continuing with TCM and waiting to start a new IVF cycle, I had a positive pregnancy test. I found out one day before going on vacation and my family doctor had booked an ultrasound for me when I would return in 12 days. We came back from our trip on a Sunday night and my ultrasound was a Monday morning. The ultrasound results left us devastated. I had a HCG of 32000, yet no baby to be found. The diagnosis: ectopic pregnancy. I had no symptoms of it being ectopic until the next day, I was taken into emergency and had surgery that resulted in a ruptured fallopian tube. I guess I had an angel looking over me because all of this unraveled after our vacation.

I decided to start seeing a fertility counselor to help me find a better coping strategy. I felt overwhelmed with losses. I had stopped going to Bikram's hot yoga due to fear of metabolic/hormonal instability. I had quit my management position and started to work part time. I stopped teaching at UBC. I avoided baby showers and actually did not attend my best friend's baby shower because I was angry and upset. I avoided family gatherings because I didn't want anyone to comment on us not having children. I avoided watching movies about babies. I started to feel depressed and anxious. I lost my carefree attitude and my happy self. I was absolutely consumed by this baby-making journey. Furthermore, I had gained so much weight and looked pregnant but had nothing to show for it.

We decided to try another IVF in February 2010 during the Vancouver Olympics. This time I produced 15 eggs resulting into 12 embryos. An error was made and only

*one embryo was transferred (it should have been two) and
it didn't work.*

*In June 2010, we tried a frozen embryo transfer with 2
embryos. I had received TCM treatment by Spence on that
day. He was so optimistic and made me feel so relaxed
that it was that treatment that remained in my mind.
Spence gave me a very positive outlook which resulted in
a positive pregnancy test at hcg 75. One week later the
test was negative. We had one more frozen embryo in the
bank but was not sure what to do.*

*During this entire time I continued with TCM because I
knew it was helping me and the embryos were looking
better and I felt better. My cramping had lessened, I was
not cold all the time anymore and I had less migraines.
Overall, I was seeing a lot of little changes that were
overlooked by western medicine. I continued with other
changes such as a gluten free diet. I stopped drinking
caffeinated beverages and any alcohol. I avoided simple
sugars and fatty foods.*

*In September 2010, we decided to switch clinics. The day
we decided to switch was an emotional roller coaster. In
the morning we had a last follow-up appointment with the
first clinic. We had lunch at a restaurant which was
surrounded by a sea of women with strollers and babies
waiting in line for a mommy-baby movie afternoon.
Daggers in my heart. In the afternoon, we met the fertility
doctor at the new clinic.*

*We tried another round of IVF which resulted in similar
outcomes but the embryos looked a lot better, not perfect
but better than before. I felt so optimistic and told myself
this was it; we were going to be pregnant! This time two
embryos were transferred but resulted in no pregnancy.
The next day I was immediately started on estrogen and
put into the frozen embryo transfer (FET) drug protocol.*

*Two more embryos were transferred and I was convinced
that it was over. I was cramping and spotting. We had no
more embryos to transfer from this round of IVF. I started
to think that maybe it just was not meant to be and I need
to just get my life back. The nurse insisted that I just go
for the pregnancy test blood work. We spent more time
trying to have a baby in our marriage than just being
married. I was completely heartbroken. I was at work and
crying in my office between seeing patients. I remember
talking to the physician I worked with and crying as I was
trying to talk about some medications. When I went back
to my office, there was a voice message saying that I had
a positive pregnancy test! What!!??? I was absolutely
shocked but very guarded at the same time because the
last time it didn't work. Well, it worked and I have a
beautiful baby girl who was born July 27, 2011! I was 33
years old when she was born.*

*We decided to try IVF after one year because I wanted
more children and I knew that this could be another long
journey. We decided to try IVF in September 2012. We
had very similar results with the same drug protocol. Two
embryos were transferred which resulted in a negative
pregnancy test. I was again immediately put into the FET
drug protocol and we decided to transfer the remaining 2
frozen embryos PLUS the one embryo from the previous
clinic, transferring a total of 3. During the thawing phase,
only one embryo survived but it was a perfect embryo. All
we needed was one baby so we remained very optimistic. I
even tried hypnotherapy to help me with this round of
FET. After this final transfer and no more frozen embryos
in the bank, we were devastated to find out that that one
did not work. At this point I was lost. I was someone who
wanted 3 children and now I only had the one. We really
thought about it and decided to prepare for just one last
round of IVF. This whole time I was so upset and just
discouraged. I was preparing myself to have acceptance
that I had one child and to just focus on her. I should be*

happy and I should just let it go.

While I was waiting for day 1 of my menstrual period to start my medications, I was getting impatient and frustrated because my period was so late! I was always on time. The first thought that came to me was, "Great! Now all of these drugs and procedures is throwing me into early menopause!" My family doctor told me to just do a home pregnancy test just to make sure. And I was shocked!! I was pregnant! I had no idea. How it could be possible?! We only had intercourse once and definitely not on an ovulating day! The fertility doctor said that this was rare but a side effect of coming off the high doses of medication. I must have had a spontaneous ovulation. I was so happy!!! I continued with TCM until the end of the first trimester.

During my second pregnancy, I found out that I had an incarcerated uterus which is very rare and my specialist had only ever seen it once before in his 30 years of practice. TCM helped with the pain and discomfort during the first trimester. I had to eventually be given an epidural when I was 15 weeks pregnant and my uterus was manually repositioned to be in my front rather than my back. I wouldn't have been able to carry full term or even past second trimester had this procedure not been completed.

On October 14, 2013, I had another beautiful and healthy baby girl.

After 32 embryos and 7 transferred, we got our second child and I could finally close this chapter of our fertility journey for good. I felt as if the shackles were removed and I wasn't a prisoner anymore. No more IVF; no more baby-making.

We have decided that we no longer wish to have any more

children; however, if it were to happen unexpectedly, then I would get my wish of having 3 children come true!

We've talked about a lot of these already but just to recap, here are 33 tips to optimize your chances of IVF success:

1. Acupuncture for both the male and female.
2. Get enough quality sleep. So important.
3. Massage therapy. Treat yourself to someone's healing touch this week; you are worth it.
4. Make sure someone has answered all your questions.
5. Divorce Dr. Google. Anyone can post on the web in seconds. You're better off heading to a book store or library and reading what the experts say.
6. Take your premium quality vitamins.
7. Schedule fun and soul-feeding activities.
8. Eat walnuts. According to TCM, they are one of the best foods to supplement reproductive strength.
9. Femoral massage. Get your partner to do this to you. It may stimulate some romance!
10. Foot soaks. Implementing a nightly routine is a must!
11. Disconnect and reconnect. Leave the mobile devices at home sometimes; you will survive.
12. Surround yourself with beauty. Be it nature or a clothing store. Whatever you find beautiful.
13. Hypnotherapy. Let someone help you go deep. You may find a release.
14. Counselling. Sometimes you just need to talk to a professional.
15. Castor oil packs. Warm that cold uterus!

16. Stress point acupressure you can do at home. With little effort, you can induce a state of calm.
17. Yoga (yin style). To all you power and hot yoga gurus out there, try Yin or Hatha.
18. Deep breathing. Without a doubt, this is the simplest and most effective thing you can do to manage stress.
19. Meditation or Qigong. Cultivate a deeper sense of awareness and consciousness.
20. Do not overeat. This is a choice that you must implement today and forever, with the possible exception for holidays.
21. Eat lots of colorful, whole, organic foods-- local when possible.
22. Laugh. Try to worry and laugh at the same time; it's impossible.
23. Slow down. If you are going too fast, you may be doing too much and not prioritizing.
24. Take a walk as slow as you can. Really, try it. No destination, take in the scenery and smell the flowers.
25. Enjoy washing your hands. A great mindfulness exercise. Smile, breathe and be grateful.
26. Eliminate coffee. You will when you are pregnant anyway; might as well start now.
27. Reduce alcohol. If it is a habit, not an occasion, this must change.
28. Eliminate dairy. Yes, eliminate. Period.
29. Eliminate junk foods. You will feel better almost instantly.
30. Drink enough quality water. Then drink a little more.
31. Avoid emotional extremes. These are based on attachment and need to be managed.
32. Stop smoking and avoid second hand

smoke.

33. Eliminate toxins from your environment. (See Step Eight).

Chapter Task:

List three positive aspects of assisted reproductive technologies (ART):

1. _____

2. _____

3. _____

Write down any questions you still have about ART:

_____

_____

_____

_____

Now go and find answers to these questions!

Step Ten

Men's Health and Well-being:

Tips for increasing male fertility

"The best relationships are partnerships."
~Rinatta Paries

For all the women who have been reading on your own so far, this will be a useful chapter for you to hand over to your male partners. We will cover the basics of how men can be their healthiest and increase the chances of having the family you both want.

Sperm is being used increasingly as a biomarker for health and potential risks to future health so the little guys are our friends and should be treated with respect.

The ideal response for a man that has been handed the diagnosis of infertility is to become accountable and take great care of himself, just as it is for women. Remember, you are half of the equation and fatherhood is no less important than motherhood.

I have been blessed with being a father to two healthy boys and I can tell you that being a dad is the best job in the world. Every day is an opportunity to show my boys a virtuous way to walk through this lifetime. That is my guiding principle for each decision I make. Having a family gives me direction and guidance, and ultimately a peace that I never thought possible. I live like each moment could be the last. I make each choice knowing my boys are watching.

These feelings are what guide my intention with the work I do each day at Yinstill. I want to help all the people that come to me start their happy, healthy families so they can share in the joy that family brings. Sometimes it takes tough love, and other times it takes gentle compassion to guide people down a better path that has a greater chance of leading to children, fulfillment and optimal health.

Male infertility affects 10% to 15% of reproductive-aged couples worldwide. Since it is so common, it is important to understand the true role it plays in male health and relationships. Men struggling with infertility suffer intense negative sexual, personal and social strains unique to this diagnosis and as a result, it can be a difficult subject to broach, so it is often ignored. There is without a doubt, the absolute need for men to be accountable. I hope the research cited in this chapter is enough to make men consider taking steps toward improvement of their own health. There is no shame in needing help getting on track with your reproductive wellness. It's no one's fault and the good news is that it's often fixable.

Semen Collection and Analysis

To begin the process of semen analysis, it must be collected in one of two ways. The first option is to ejaculate into a sterile container, but because masturbation on demand is not easy, it may take some mental preparation and may be less preferable than option two. This method is most conveniently performed in the facility provided at the laboratory.

The second option is to be sent away with a special condom that can be brought back at a later time. Collection at home is acceptable provided the sample is transported within one hour and kept at body temperature.

This may also be the preference of men that are prohibited by religious or personal practices that do not permit masturbation. Semen should never be collected in an ordinary condom, however, as they contain substances that kill sperm.

It should be noted that it is important to refrain from ejaculation for 2-4 days before the sample is required and that semen collected by interrupted intercourse is not favoured since it risks the loss of sample, particularly the first fraction of the ejaculate.

If sperm parameters come back as abnormal, I recommend men going to a local fertility clinic to get a more accurate and thorough semen analysis done as often times, busy community labs do not do their analysis within the recommended time limit of sixty minutes. This can have negative effects on outcome measures. A urine sample after ejaculation is also a good idea to check for retrograde ejaculation.

Intracytoplasmic Sperm Injection (ICSI)
An advanced method of IVF, this is a procedure in which one sperm is extracted with a syringe, and injected into an egg, therefore eliminating the need for the sperm to penetrate the egg itself, as in regular IVF. Because of the existence of this procedure, even when semen parameters do not fall within normal lab ranges, men are often told things are fine because many medical professionals believe that ICSI makes the negative impact of poor sperm irrelevant. I believe that everything possible should be done to improve the semen parameters before simply jumping into ICSI. To some degree, poor sperm quality has to be a reflection of overall health and whenever possible, should be addressed before becoming a parent.

NOTE: *Doctors should be informed of any illness that has happened in the last three months since it takes 100*

Dr. Spence Pentland

days for sperm to mature and problems at any time in the last 3 months could affect the semen sample.

Causes of Male Factor Infertility

* It is worth spending the extra money to have your tests done at a fertility lab, or a lab specifically for male testing. Regular labs that do not understand the importance of accuracy and timing and may disregard seemingly insignificant details that are, in fact, very telling.

* It is worth doing more than one test because semen results can vary a lot depending on factors like stress, illness etc.

* The appearance of normal semen should be opalescent and grayish. Yellowish semen may show high intakes of vitamin supplements, abstinence or jaundice. An infection may show some red in the semen.

Before we can address an issue, we need to know what it is. While many problems with sperm are of unknown cause, here are some we do know about:

● Undescended testis - Usually detected and corrected soon after birth. If this is left untreated for very long, it can have negative effects on fertility.

● Testicular trauma - This could affect overall testicular function or the damage could breach the blood-testis barrier which can introduce antisperm antibodies into the

228

reproductive tract making it difficult for the sperm to swim.

- Hormonal - An imbalance of the hormones necessary for proper sperm production and sexual function is common. Either the messages that the brain is sending to the testes is deficient or is being blocked, or there is a problem with the functioning of the testes so the brain is trying to compensate by sending out more and more hormones.
- Klinefelter's - A somewhat rare genetic disorder resulting in an extra female X chromosome. This often manifests as enhanced female characteristics like enlarged breast tissue and reduced muscle mass.
- Mumps - A disease that if caught in childhood can affect fertility in men.
- Varicocele - Abnormal enlargement of the scrotal veins that drain the testis, which creates Heat and may adversely affect sperm production.
- Absence of vas deferens - This is often due to cystic fibrosis, a genetic disorder. This makes it impossible for sperm to travel from the testis to the penis for ejaculation.
- Medications & steroids - Antihypertensives, anti-inflammatories, antihistamines.
- Toxins in our environment -Toxins in our environment can mimic estrogen and throw off hormonal balance. Many common substances have shown detrimental effects on fertility. To read more about this, visit Step Seven: Toxin Awareness.
- Radiation or chemotherapy - Cancer treatments can adversely affect sperm. Freezing sperm in men of reproductive age prior to treatments is often standard policy as a result.
- Infrared saunas - I have seen these drop sperm counts to zero. Heat may very well be the #1 enemy of sperm.

- Thyroid issues - Just like in women, the thyroid should be balanced before conception. Both hypo or hyper may have effects on various sperm parameters.
- Obesity - Plenty of research confirms that being overweight negatively impacts male fertility. This may also predispose their children to difficulties with weight, diabetes and other metabolic conditions.
- Blue collar careers - A higher percentage of blue collar workers (skilled or unskilled manual labour) report poor semen parameters when compared with white collar workers (professional, managerial, or administrative work). This was one of many factors identified by researchers from Women's Hospital in Heidelberg, Germany (Gerhard et al , 1992).
- Mobile phones - Much like the cigarette, it's our new bad habit. Even while not in use, if it's sitting beside your testicles, it could be impacting the health of your sperm.
- Tight pants or underwear - Heat being the #1 enemy of sperm tells us that tight synthetic garments should be left on the rack.
- Genetic abnormalities - Karyotype problems or Y-microdeletion problems. Simply put, these are issues with the number (deletions), appearance and proper positioning of chromosomes. The most common being Klinefelter's discussed above.
- Heat extremes - Environmental heat like that experienced by chefs, or internally generated heat caused by fevers.
- Surgery - Lower abdominal surgery such as with inguinal hernia has the potential to break the blood-testis barrier resulting in the formation of antisperm antibodies, a condition where antibodies attach to the sperm and inhibit its ability to swim.
- Bad habits -Alcohol, nicotine, marijuana, cocaine

and any other recreational drugs may have negative effects on sperm and overall health.

- Poor diet - This links intimately to obesity, as well as the potential negative impacts that paternal nutrition may have on offspring. Read on for more details on a sperm-friendly diet.

AntiSperm Antibodies

A man may produce antibodies to his own sperm, which means that the immune system is mounting an attack against his own sperm.

For the most part, sperm is protected from the immune system by the 'blood-testis barrier', but when this barrier is breached (often in sloppy inguinal hernia operations), antisperm antibodies are formed and the immune system attacks, like it would to any other foreign invader. There are also theories that infection and inflammation may potentially cause a 'leakage' in this barrier, or early sperm cells, which begin their life on the immune side of this barrier, and for unknown reasons alert the immune response. Regardless of the cause, antisperm antibodies most often affect the sperms ability to optimally swim to its destination, as the extra weight of its passengers (the antibodies attached to it) slow it down.

From a Chinese medical perspective, antisperm antibodies often present in men with Dampness and Heat. This could translate into infection, inflammation, constitutional predisposition to these patterns, or a result of poor lifestyle choices such as greasy foods, alcohol and not enough rest. I also find that these men have a tendency toward allergies and sensitivities to foods and their environment. This tells me that their immune system needs regulation and their presenting TCM patterns need to be rectified.

Dr. Spence Pentland

Research with Chinese herbal medicine has shown better results versus treatment with steroids to suppress the immune system (see references below in Chinese herbal medicine section). In my personal practice, I have seen a reduction in ASA in many male clients when treated diligently with Chinese herbal medicine for a period of at least 3-6 months.

Semen Analysis

This next bit of information is somewhat technical but it will empower those of you that thrive on science. For those of you that find the medical jargon confusing, feel free to read ahead.

- *Normozoospermia* - An ejaculate falling within normal range of parameters.
- *Liquefaction* - Semen should liquefy within 15-60 minutes (with 15 minutes being the norm).
- *Appearance* - Normal semen is opalescent and grayish. Yellowish semen may show high intakes of vitamin supplements, abstinence or jaundice. An infection may show some red in the semen.
- *Volume* - Total volume can range from 1-5ml. Too much can mean it is diluted. Low volume may show past infection blocking the tubes, retrograde ejaculation, or problems with accessory glands such as the seminal vesicles or the prostate. Sometimes there is an absence of the vas deferens. Volume drops 20% between 30 and 50 years of age. (Aspermia = no ejaculate).
- *Agglutination* - Higher amounts of agglutination (sperm sticking together) point to antiSperm antibodies and can affect motility by coating the sperm and bind to cervical mucus preventing proper movement and difficulty fertilizing the egg. This is common in men who have had reproductive tract surgery.

232

- *Motility* - Rapid progressive motile swimmers are really all that matter when it comes to conception and ability to penetrate the egg. This is not distinguished in community labs - even twitching non-progressive sperm are factored into a motile %. At least 32% should be progressive (the higher the percentage of rapid progressive the better). Motility decreases by 3.1% per year. (Asthenozoospermia = low motility). Sperm DNA fragmentation should be noted here.
- *Concentration* - There should be at least 15 million sperm per ml of semen. Caffeine, tobacco, alcohol, drugs, diet, exercise and stress can also affect this. If it is very low, there may be a genetic chromosomal defect. (Oligozoospermia = sperm concentration of less than 15 million).
- *Count* - >39 million. This is total sperm count per ejaculate. (concentration X volume (ml) = count). Count drops nearly 5% per year. (Azoospermia = no spermatozoa in the ejaculate).
- *Morphology* - At least 4% of the sperm in a semen sample should be shaped normally. Avoiding things that are toxic to sperm are very important with morphology. (Teratozoospermia = poor morphology).
- *Acidity* - Semen has a pH between 7.2 and 8.
- *Round Cell Concentration* - Immature sperm or white blood cells. Too many of these in a sample may indicate infection.
- *Sperm DNA fragmentation* - The structural integrity of the DNA within the sperm may be associated with miscarriage (*see 'sperm and miscarriage' section) and diminished fertility. As a result of testing for this semen parameter being expensive, research has attempted to correlate more common semen parameters with DNA fragmentation. In a retrospective study of over 1000 men, data indicated that poor motility is the

sperm parameter abnormality most closely related to sperm DNA damage. Therefore, we can hypothesize that if we can treat and improve sperm motility, DNA fragmentation rates may also improve (*Belloc, 2014*).

*WHO standards 2010 can be viewed at - http://whqlibdoc.who.int/publications/2010/97892415477 89_eng.pdf?ua=1

Diet and Nutrition

> *"How am I going to live today in order to create the tomorrow I'm committed to?"* ~Tony Robbins

Step Five is a great resource for diet information and how it relates to fertility as well as TCM, but here we will talk about some specific sperm-friendly foods and how best to incorporate them.

Folic Acid

Two studies conducted in the Netherlands emphasized the importance of folic acid for healthy sperm.

The first study, published in The Journal of Andrology, emphasized the importance of B6, folate (B9, folic acid), B12 and homocysteine levels in the production of sperm (*Boxmeer et al, 2007*).

The second, published in Fertility and Sterility, had a similar result stating that low concentrations of folate (folic acid, B9) in seminal plasma may be detrimental for sperm DNA stability (*Boxmeer et al, 2009*).

So how can you boost the folic acid in your diet? As referenced on the *Dieticians of Canada* website (dietitians.ca), dark green vegetables like broccoli and spinach and dried legumes such as chickpeas, beans and lentils are good natural sources of folate (folic acid). The best sources of Vitamin B12 include eggs, meat, fish and poultry, and the top sources of Vitamin B6 are liver, wild Atlantic salmon, tuna and fortified meatless alternatives.

Sarah Kimmins, an expert in epigenetics and reproduction, has published many articles emphasizing the importance of the father-to-be diet. The study focused on a diet deficient in folate and found excellent motivation for men to adhere to a folate-rich diet.

A father's diet before conception can affect the health of his offspring. There's a common perception that the father can do whatever he wants without consequence to others. Kimmins research shows that this isn't the case — men really need to think carefully about the life they're living because future generations can be impacted.

The researchers examined the sperm of males with a folate deficient diet, and found genetic links to development of diseases such as cancer, diabetes, autism and schizophrenia. They also found a link between a father's diet and possible muscular and skeletal birth defects (*Kimmins, 2013*).

Lycopene and Carotene

In a study published in Fertility & Sterility, a prominent peer reviewed medical journal, positive correlations between the intake of the antioxidant lycopene and sperm morphology (shape), and the antioxidant carotene and sperm motility (movement) (*Zareba, 2013*) were found. As talked about in the Step on diet, adding color is always encouraged.

Here are some examples of lycopene and carotene rich foods:

- Lycopene Rich Foods for Sperm Morphology: Tomatoes (sun dried are best, raw and cooked are also good), guava, watermelon, grapefruit, parsley, basil, asparagus, liver, red cabbage.

- Carotene Rich Foods for Sperm Motility: Sweet potato, kale, carrots, greens (spinach, mustard, turnip, collard), butternut squash, red leaf lettuce.

Protein

Men need to make sure they are getting enough protein. This is not an issue for most men, but for some it can be. If you are a vegetarian or vegan and are having trouble conceiving, TCM would advise you to begin including some animal or fish protein in your diet. Get as much as you can from fish and vegetable sources but a good quality steak (happy cattle only, please) can be medicinal. It shouldn't be a large part of a man's diet because cholesterol levels should also be paid close attention to but consider it an augmentation.

A good rule of thumb - if it is bad for your heart, it is bad for your sperm and balance is always good. Certain foods, such as fish, will combat cholesterol so the more fish you eat, the more fatty four-legged animal muscle you can have.

And speaking of four-legged animals...

In a study of bulls, the conclusion published in the Journal of Animal Science stated that plant-based diets reduced the amount of fructose in the semen samples of the bulls being observed (*Shirley, 1963*). Fructose is a simple sugar present in semen necessary to feed the sperm so that their mitochondria can produce ATP (cellular energy). Sperm needs this sugar to get the energy required to whip their tail so they can swim.

Alcohol

If you are healthy and your sperm shows no abnormalities, then two or three drinks once or twice a week should be okay. But while you are trying to conceive a child, giving up alcohol for a while certainly wouldn't hurt. If your sperm *does* show abnormalities or you have a reproductive hormone imbalance, I would definitely recommend abstaining from alcohol.

Recommended Supplements

Zinc
A study done in two fertility practices in the Netherlands showed a 74% increase in total normal sperm count after combined zinc sulfate (66mg) and folic acid (5mg) treatment for 26 weeks (6 months) in both subfertile and fertile men (*Wong et al, 2002*).
Vitamin B6, B9 (folate), B12 Homocysteine blends
See page 209 for expansion on these and how to incorporate them into your diet.

CoQ10 & L-Carnitine
Research in Japan on 212 men with poor semen parameters of unknown cause were given either 300mg of CoQ10 or a placebo for 6 months (106 men in each group). Coenzyme Q10 supplementation resulted in a statistically significant improvement in sperm concentration, motility and morphology, as well as a positive effect on reproductive hormone levels (Safarinejad, 2009).
- Recent research done in Iran also showed improvement in semen parameters and reproductive hormone levels (*Ghanbarzadeh, 2013*).
- Another study involving men with low motility showed that taking 200mg CoQ10 for 6 months significantly improved this condition (*Balercia et*

al, 2009).

<u>*Fish Oils high in Omega 3 EPA and DHA*</u>

- 238 infertile men with poor sperm count, motility and morphology were randomised to eicosapentaenoic (EPA) and docosahexaenoic acids (DHA), 1.84 g per day, or placebo for 32 weeks. Significant improvement in semen parameters was noted in the EPA DHA group. The researchers concluded that men with low levels of EPA and DHA may benefit from omega-3 FA supplementation (Safarinejad, 2011).
- Research from Virginia published in Theriogenology - An International Journal of Animal Reproduction showed an increase in the amount of sperm per ejaculation in boars that were supplemented with Omega-3 (*Estienne, 2000*).
- A study published in the Journal of Clinical Nutrition showed that infertile men had lower

Alcohol and Fertility

In a 2005 paper, 'Effect of chronic alcoholism on male fertility hormones and semen quality' (Muthusami et al, 2005,), it concluded that chronic alcohol consumption (2-3 drinks per day, 5 days per week) lowered testosterone levels, raised estrogen levels and significantly decreased all semen parameters.

concentrations of Omega-3 than fertile men. These results suggest that more research should be performed to assess the potential benefits of Omega-3 supplementation as a therapeutic approach in infertile men (*Safarinejad, 2010*).

<u>*Probiotics (i.e. acidophilus, bifidum)*</u>
Aid the body in digesting and absorbing nutrition for

sperm health, producing B vitamins (see the importance of B6, B9, B12 above), and immune regulation possibly playing an important role with immune infertility conditions such as antisperm antibodies.

Vitamin D
A Japanese study displayed the importance of the role of Vitamin D in male reproductive health. It indicated that Vitamin D deficiencies resulted in decreased sperm count and decreased motility (*Kinuta et al, 2000*).

Multivitamin
These will cover minimum nutritional requirements of anything that may be missing in your diet.

Obesity

The Aberdeen Fertility Centre at the University of Aberdeen revealed that obese men produced 60% less seminal fluid than men with a healthy Body Mass Index and had 40% higher levels of abnormal sperm. The study also found that severely underweight men, with a Body Mass Index less than 19, also had poorer sperm quality than men in the healthy weight range. Speaking at the European Society of Human Reproduction and Embryology meeting in Barcelona, Dr. Ghiyath Shayeb, who led the study, said obese men could improve their sperm quality by losing weight and achieving a healthy BMI (*Shayeb, 2011*).

A multicenter study published in the pages of 'Fertility and Sterility' showed that embryos from obese male mice had reduced cleavage and decreased development to blastocyst (define) stage during IVF culture relative to males of normal BMI. Blastocysts from obese males implanted at a reduced rate, and the proportion of fetuses that developed was significantly decreased (Mitchell, 2011).

NOTE: *BMI or Body Mass Index is a measure of relative weight based on an individual's mass and height.*

Stress and its Effects on Male Fertility

In my clinical practice, it is abundantly clear that the management of stress plays a significant role in optimizing fertility.

There is a growing body of evidence that correlates psychological stress such as anxiety and depression to reproductive hormonal imbalance, production of subfertile sperm and poor IVF outcomes.

Regularly I see this type of research confirmed but after an acupuncture session, men leave the clinic with a sense of calm. They tell me that it provides an overall sense of well-being, which is reflected in all aspects of their life from relationships to increased productivity and better sleep.

Studies

- Anxiety and depression lower testosterone levels and correlate with poor semen quality (*Bhongade et al., 2014*).
- Men who have difficulty describing their feelings present with lower sperm concentration (*De Gennaro, 2003*).
- Stressful life events may be associated with decreased semen quality in fertile men (*Gollenberg, 2010*).
- Increased levels of anxiety were associated with lower semen volume, sperm concentration and count, reduced sperm motility and increased sperm DNA fragmentation of IVF patients (Vellani, 2013).
- Sperm concentration and motility decreased when

comparing prior semen samples to samples given on egg retrieval day during IVF (*Clark, 1998*).

- Men with insomnia were tested to have poorer quality sperm and smaller testi size than men who sleep well (*Jensen, 2012*).
- Men who experienced two or more stressful life events in the past year compared with no stressful events had a lower percentage of motile sperm and a lower percentage of morphologically normal sperm (Janevic, 2014).

Stress has a negative impact on all aspects of health and male fertility is no exception. It is important to find ways to manage stress. For some ideas, refer to Step Four under the heading of stress.

NOTE: *In a recent study conducted on mice, it was revealed that acupuncture regulates the specific hormones associated with the biochemical reactions that take place in the body as a result of stress.*

This study demonstrated that acupuncture provides a sense of balance rather than simply suppression of the stress response. The resulting effect is a greater ability to manage and react to stress (Wang, 2014).

TCM and Male Infertility

Often a TCM doctor specializing in the treatment of male factor infertility is the only healthcare professional that men have a chance to really talk with since few healthcare practitioners are well versed in both the mind and body aspects of male factor infertility.

It is rewarding to connect with my male patients and give them the emotional support needed as well as treatment and tools to improve their overall health, well-being and fertility.

Treatment is intended to improve chances of natural conception, IVF success and reduce the incidence of miscarriage. In addition to improving semen parameters, TCM addresses issues that may directly affect fertility such as impotence, premature ejaculation and low libido, as well as helping with stress, aches and pains, and many other ailments men typically suffer from that may be impeding fertility. These include urinary and prostate issues, hypertension, anger and irritability and digestive or bowel conditions.

Acupuncture

As detailed in Step One, a TCM treatment plan includes acupuncture and/or herbal medicine and is individually engineered to increase overall health and fertility. Recommended treatment should be through at least 1-2 full cycles of spermatogenesis (the production or development of mature sperm). 12-24 acupuncture sessions once or twice a week, within a 3-6 month period.

The following statements are conclusions of various studies showing the positive effects on sperm with Chinese herbal medicine and acupuncture.

- 82 infertile men who achieved a poor fertilization rate in at least 2 IVF/ICSI cycles were given acupuncture twice per week for 8 weeks then did another IVF/ICSI. The fertilization rates after acupuncture (66.2%) were significantly higher than that before treatment (40.2%), (*Zhang, 2002*).

- For the following pilot study, a group of 32 infertile men with abnormal semen analysis were randomly divided into two groups; one group was given 10 acupuncture treatments over 5 weeks, and the other, no treatment. Significant improvements were demonstrated in the acupuncture group compared to the control group, in particular improved motility and morphology (*Siterman, 1997*).

- This pilot study showed a positive effect of acupuncture on sperm count, but this time on men with such low sperm counts (or no sperm) that they would usually require a testicular biopsy to extract sperm for use in an IVF cycle. Seven of the 15 men with no sperm at all produced sperm detectable by the light microscope after a course of 10 acupuncture treatments, i.e., enough sperm could be produced for ICSI to be performed without recourse to testicular biopsy. The control group with similar semen analysis and no treatment showed no change after three months. It should also be noted that males with genital tract inflammation exhibited the most remarkable improvement in sperm density (*Siterman, 2000*).

- In this study involving 80 men, the effects of abdominal electroacupuncture (acupuncture in which the needles used carry a mild electric current) improved testicular blood flow was shown. Just as electroacupuncture can increase blood flow to the ovaries and uterus, it can as well to the testicles. These researchers suggest that such a stimulus may address the damaged microcirculation associated with varicoceles, and with aging. They note that decreased testicular arterial blood flow may result in impaired spermatogenesis from defective metabolism in the microcirculatory bed (*Cakmak, 2008*).

- In this prospective, randomized, single-blind, placebo-controlled study, 28 infertile patients with poor motility and low count received acupuncture twice weekly for 6 weeks according to the principles of traditional Chinese medicine and 29 infertile patients received placebo acupuncture. A significantly higher percentage of motile (moving) sperm was shown and the authors conclude that the results of the present study support the significance of acupuncture in male patients with low sperm motility (*Dieterle, 2009*).

- 28 male factor infertility patients received acupuncture twice a week over a period of 5 weeks. The samples from the treatment group were randomized with semen samples from the untreated control group. A general improvement of sperm quality, specifically in the ultrastructural integrity of sperm, was seen after acupuncture. The researchers concluded that male infertility could benefit from employing acupuncture (*Pei, 2005*).

- Men that manifest low sperm count and higher scrotal temperatures due to genital tract inflammation or poor lifestyle habits can benefit from the scrotal temperature lowering effects of acupuncture (*Siterman, 2009*).

Chinese Herbal Medicine

- Protective effects of Hochuekkito (a combination of 10 raw Japanese herbs) on sperm was found on sperm with antisperm antibodies (ASA). Although normal sperm with ASA was used in this report, since the sperm of infertile patients are said to be more fragile, this results imply that direct protective effect is one of the mechanism of Hochuekkito for male infertility (*Yamanaka, 1998*).

- 156 men with low sperm count and inability to conceive were administered individually modified

244

versions of the Chinese herbal formula, Sheng Jing Qiang You Tang (Engender Essence & Strengthen Fertility Decoction) for 3-6 months. They were not allowed to drink alcohol, smoke or have sex. In 98 men, their sperm count increased above WHO standards, and 35 men showed an increase in sperm count but did not yet meet 'fertile' WHO criteria (*Zhang, 2005*).

- 100 men with low sperm count and poor sperm motility were treated with individually modified Chinese herbal formulations combined with Clomid and Vitamin E daily for 15-60 days (37.3 days average). 82% showed significant increases in both count and motility. This may be a viable treatment option for men with poor sperm motility and low sperm counts (*Chang-Jie, 2007*).

- 100 cases of male immune infertility in the treatment group were treated with Yikang Decoction, while 100 cases were treated with prednisone (steroid used for immune suppression) as the controls. The Yikang Decoction has a more stable effect for male immune infertility than prednisone. Antisperm antibodies, percentage of motile sperm, pregnancy rates and sperm agglutination (clumping) were all significantly better in the group treated with the Chinese herbal formula, Yikang Decoction vs the prednisone treatment group (*Sun, 2006*).

- 132 men with antisperm antibodies were treated for 1.5-4.5 months with a Chinese herbal formula, Ju He Wan. After treatment, 120 men (91%) tested negative for antisperm antibodies (compared to only 45% of the group treated with prednisone). 74 of these same men conceived after 1.5-3 months of treatment (*Cheng, 2007*).

- The effects of a Chinese herb, Cornus officinalis, on the motility of human sperm was studied. A water-based extract was prepared from the dried fruits of the herb and used in this study. The crude extract showed substantial stimulatory effects on sperm motility (*Jeng, 1997*).

- Mice taking Tai-bao Chinese herbal medicine displayed significantly higher rates of implantation and pregnancy, as well as comparative rates of lowering effects of antisperm antibodies as prednisone controls. Chinese medicine Tai-bao possesses a regulatory effect on reproductive immune function, inhibitory effect on antisperm cytotoxic antibody, and promoting effect on pregnancy (*Lai, 1997*).

- 87 cases of male infertility were treated with Bu Shen Sheng Jing Pill, and the comprehensive semen routine analysis score was enhanced significantly. The result showed that this prescription had a regulatory function in follicle stimulating hormone, luteotropic hormone, testosterone and cortisol (could bring the enhanced or reduced hormone level back to normal range), (*Yue, 1996*).

- 37 infertile men with varicocele were treated with Guizhi-Fuling-Wan for at least 3 months. Before and after the administration, semen qualities such as sperm concentration and motility were examined, and the varicocele was graded. A varicocele disappearance rate of 80% was obtained with 40 out of 50 varicocele, and improvement of sperm concentration and motility were found in 71.4% and 62.1% of patients, respectively. From these results, Guizhi-Fuling-Wan is considered to be effective for circulation disorders in varicocele as well as semen quality (*Ishikawa, 1996*).

- 90 men with immune infertility were selected and randomly divided into two groups; 60 in the treatment group treated by Huzhangdanshenyin, and the other 30 in the control, treated by prednisone, both for three months. The improvement of clinical symptoms, immunologic indexes (antisperm antibodies in serum and seminal plasma) and sperm indexes (semen liquefied duration, motility, viability, density and abnormal morphology rate) were observed and the results analyzed. The Chinese medicine Huzhangdanshenyin works more effectively than prednisone in the treatment of male immune infertility. It could improve the antisperm antibody reversing ratio, clinical symptoms and signs and ameliorate sperm indexes with no obvious adverse effects (*Lu, 2006*).

According to TCM, male factor infertility can be categorized into the following three disease mechanisms: Blockage, Deficiency and Heat.

In my experience, the clinical picture is a varied combination of patterns that may span all three of these mechanisms.

Blockage is most often caused by Qi Stagnation, Dampness, Phlegm, Heat and Blood Stasis. Deficiencies are most often a result of insufficient Yin, Yang, Qi and/or Blood. Finally, the generation of Heat is a result of any chronic blockage or more advanced Yin deficiency. Again, it is important to note that every patient will exhibit at least two or more of the patterns below simultaneously but in varying degrees. For example, a man may clearly fit into the pattern of Damp Heat but may also show signs of Blood Stasis and Qi Stagnation. Therefore, it is important to rank yourself (or your husband) in presenting order so that recommendations that are most relevant can be prioritized for implementation. It is equally important that a licensed TCM doctor determines the precise pattern differentiation before Chinese herbal medicine or more extensive treatment is administered.

Let's have a look at some of the patterns so you can see where you may fit.

Qi Stagnation (causing Heat)

Causes: Anger in all its forms including impatience, irritability, frustration, sarcasm, road rage, etc. is among the primary causes. Stress is a close second and can be characterized as any emotional extreme, sexual anxiety, the feeling of being stuck or unfulfilled, lack of joy and work/life pressures. Physical activity, either extreme or deficient, may both cause the Qi to stagnate. Also any trauma to the lower abdomen or genitals.

Symptoms: Bowel movements alternating from loose to constipated, neck tension, shallow breathing, frequent sighing or yawning, possible digestive issues, a wiry pulse (feels like a guitar string snapping against your fingers). Tongue body may be purplish or have orangey sides.

Andrology: May display as low sperm count, low motility, poor morphology, low volume, delayed liquefaction, often see erectile dysfunction, difficult and/or premature ejaculation, difficult to achieve orgasm, low libido.

Diet: Please refer to Step Five for TCM pattern specific dietary recommendations.

Supplements: Coq10, fish oil high in EPA, homocysteine (B6,folate,12), antioxidants, digestive enzymes (between meals), probiotics, zinc, Vitamin D. Properly prescribed Chinese herbal medicine works extremely well for this pattern. *See Step Five for full information.

Lifestyle recommendations: Sleep in and wear natural breathable fibers like linens or cotton. If anger or any of the above mentioned emotions are prevalent in your character, getting help to control them is important. Try to set aside time for relaxation. Meditation, Qigong, Tai Chi, or Yoga would be excellent activities to restore balance and reduce stress.

Damp Heat

Causes: Sedentary lifestyle, poor dietary habits such as over consumption of alcohol, greasy foods and sweets. Damp or hot climate, synthetic underwear and pants, professions that are exposed to excessive heat such as welders or chefs, stress and digestive issues.

Symptoms: Itchy and/or warm sweaty groin, genitals and anus, skin eruptions in groin and buttocks area, scanty warm yellow urine, fullness in lower abdomen, gas and bloating, fatigue, anxiety, thirst for cool fluids, bowel movements may be accompanied by an unfinished feeling. Tongue can be sticky with a thick yellow coat especially at the root and a red body is not uncommon. Pulse is often rapid.

Andrology: May display as low sperm count, poor morphology, low volume, low motility, antisperm antibodies, semen appears yellowish, may see white blood cells in semen, varicocele.

Diet: Please refer to Step Five for TCM pattern specific dietary recommendations.

Supplements: Fiber, probiotics, fish oil high in EPA, homocysteine (B6,9,12), antioxidants, broad spectrum digestive enzymes (between meals), zinc, CoQ10, Vitamin D. Properly prescribed Chinese herbal medicine works extremely well for this pattern. See Step Five for full information.

Lifestyle recommendations: Sleep with and wear natural breathable fibers like linen and cotton. Keep your genitals cool by giving them lots of fresh air time, set aside time for relaxation, express gratitude and find ways to cultivate spiritual well-being. Excessive cycling is not recommended. Avoid triggers that may cause alcohol consumption and poor dietary choices. Some men may need to simply take things down a notch, as the fast-paced life they are leading is causing Damp Heat and negatively affecting their sperm.

Kidney Yang Deficiency

Causes: Advanced Paternal Age (APA), hypothyroidism, excessive physical work for many years, constitutional weakness as a genetic predisposition, chronic back and knee injuries, long term fear, excessive exposures to cold, and over consumption of antibiotics or other medications.

Symptoms: Overweight, swollen, pale, fatigued, slow moving, weak, cold (particularly in the limbs), affinity for heat, aversion to cold, listless, fatigued, lack of spirit, pale white complexion, cold damp sensation in the external reproductive organs, copious clear urine, nocturia (urination at night), lack of power, will, or assertion that propels and targets the major episodes of life, fear, paralyzed by the unknown, passive, lack ability to assert themselves, easily controlled by others, take blame, feel guilty, large sense of responsibility, sexual anxiety. Tongue may be pale and swollen with white moist coat.

May all worsen with excessive sexual activity.

Andrology: Low sperm count and motility, rapid liquefaction, clear in appearance, premature ejaculation, weak orgasm and ejaculation, tired and/or dizzy after ejaculation, low libido, may see erectile dysfunction.

Diet: Please refer to Step Five for TCM pattern specific dietary recommendations.

Supplements: Whole food multivitamin, probiotics, CoQ10, fish oil high in EPA, antioxidants, homocysteine (B6,9,12), zinc, Vitamin D. Long term administration of Chinese herbal medicine is often necessary to improve Kidney deficiency. See Step Five for full information.

Lifestyle recommendations: Keeping warm and not allowing your body to become cold is important. Finding a fitness routine that builds strength and focuses on aerobic activity, getting enough sleep, managing stress, socializing with other men, seeking help if depression is an issue, eliminating alcohol, tobacco and marijuana, losing weight if necessary, finding help in overcoming your fears and building confidence and avoiding toxins in our environment that mimic estrogen.

Kidney Yin/Essence Deficiency (causing Heat)

Causes: Constitutional weakness due to a genetic predisposition and/or 'burning the candle at both ends' via excessive work, play, exercise or a busy life without proper attention given to adequate nutrition and rest. This is also a common pattern in those which use their minds a lot, such as students and academics.

Symptoms: These people tend to be thin or emaciated, have red cheeks, be restless, quick moving with narrow shoulders, weak lower knees, tinnitus (ringing in ears), insomnia, warm hands and feet, night sweats, hot flushes, dryness of mouth and skin, dry stools, anxiety and irritability. They are fidgety, jumpy, lack tranquility are fearful and have sexual anxiety and diminished willpower. Tongue is red with a thin scanty coating that is white or yellowish, and the pulse feels rapid.

Andrology: No sperm in ejaculate, poor count morphology and volume, delayed liquefaction, thick sticky semen that may appear yellowish (if Heat is present), may see premature ejaculation.

Diet: Please refer to Step Five for TCM pattern specific dietary recommendations.

Supplements: Whole food multivitamin, probiotics, CoQ10, fish oil high in EPA, antioxidants, homocysteine (B6,9,12), zinc, Vitamin D. Long term administration of Chinese herbal medicine is often necessary to improve kidney deficiency. See Step Five for full information.

Lifestyle recommendations: Relaxation, sleep and rest are all very important. Reducing work and exercise may be necessary. Sleep with and wear natural breathable fibers. Incorporate deep breathing into daily activities. Meditation, Qigong, Tai Chi, or Yoga would be excellent activities to restore balance.

Qi and Blood Deficiency

Causes: Excessive physical work for many years, constitutional weakness due to a genetic predisposition, poor nutrition, chronic depression, sadness or worry, recovery from injury or illness, lack of exercise.

Symptoms: Fatigue, low energy, a weak immune system, pale complexion, digestive issues such as bloating and gas, loose bowel movements, listlessness, lack of spirit, heart palpitations, difficulty falling asleep, poor memory, dizziness, poor appetite, laziness, shortness of breath, pale nails, brittle hair, the tongue body is pale, the pulse feels deep, thin and soft. Prone to worry, over-thinking, stress, chronic illness, poor self-esteem and lack of motivation.

Andrology: Low sperm count, low motility, low volume, diluted appearance (watery), may present with erectile dysfunction, premature ejaculation and low libido, varicocele.

Diet: Please refer to Step Five for TCM pattern specific dietary recommendations.

Supplements: Whole food multivitamin, probiotics, CoQ10, fish oil high in EPA, antioxidants, zinc, Vitamin D. See Step Five for full information.

Lifestyle recommendations: Focus on a fitness routine that builds strength and focuses on aerobic activity. Get enough sleep, manage stress, schedule social time. Seek help if depression is an issue, eliminate alcohol, tobacco and marijuana, lose weight if necessary. Find help in overcoming your fears and building confidence and avoid toxins in our environment that mimic estrogen. See Step Seven for more on this.

Blood Stasis

Causes: Any chronic health imbalance or TCM pattern including poor lifestyle habits, over time will eventually result in Blood Stasis. Other causes may include trauma or surgery.

Symptoms: Fixed pain anywhere on the body that is stabbing in character, chronic disease history, purple lips, spider veins, dull grey face. The tongue may be purple in color and/or may have purple spots and sublingual veins that are dark and distended. The pulse has a choppy nature, not feeling like it passes smoothly under the fingers and may vary in rate.

Andrology: Low sperm count, motility and volume. Poor morphology, the presence of antisperm antibodies, possible red blood cells in semen, also may present with erectile dysfunction, pain with ejaculation, pain in the testis or scrotum and varicocele.

Diet: Please refer to Step Five for TCM pattern specific dietary recommendations.

Supplements: Fish oil high in EPA, homocysteine (B6,9,12), CoQ10. See Step Five for full information.

Lifestyle recommendations: Cardio training for ½ hour 4 times per week. Daily stretching is very important. Deep breathing incorporated into daily activities.

Phlegm

Causes: Poor diet, i.e., excessive consumption of greasy and sweet foods, overeating in general, alcohol, sedentary lifestyle, chronic sadness and high stress levels, worry, overthinking, hypothyroidism, low testosterone and repeated use of over-the-counter cold medications and/or antibiotics.

Symptoms: Foggy mind, chest oppression, nausea, dizziness, lack of coordination, sinusitis, snoring, copious sputum, palpitations, overweight, centralized obesity (aka a beer belly). The tongue will appear swollen with a thick slippery greasy coating.

Andrology: Low sperm count, volume and motility, poor morphology. May see erectile dysfunction, possible ejaculation difficulty, low libido, may see testicle pain including hardness lumps or swelling. May be present with enlarged prostate and accompanied symptoms such as urinary difficulty including dribbling, pain, frequency and reduced flow.

Diet: Please refer to Step Five for TCM pattern specific dietary recommendations.

Supplements: Fiber, broad spectrum digestive enzymes (with meals), probiotics, CoQ10, fish oil high in EPA, antioxidants, zinc, Vitamin D. See Step Five for full information.

Lifestyle recommendations: Physical focus should be on aerobic exercise to burn fat. Try jogging for ½ hour 4 times per week.

A few suggestions everyone can benefit from:

- *Jump on a rebound trampoline for 10 minutes each day.*
- *Contribute to your community.*
- *Prioritize your life and spend little time doing things that will not take you closer to your dreams and goals.*
- *Avoid spending time with people who trigger your bad habits.*
- *Express gratitude for what you have.*
- *Find ways to cultivate spiritual well-being.*

Dr. Spence Pentland

Sperm and Miscarriage

"The most important thing a father can do for his children is to love their mother." ~Theodore Hesburgh

Being half the genetic code, there is a strong possibility that poor sperm quality plays a role in miscarriage, yet in my experience this potential link is never spoken about or tested for, even in recurrent loss clinics. I believe this is mostly due to the lack of medical treatment for poor sperm. ICSI (intracytoplasmic sperm injection) may help sidestep the issue of DNA fragmentation, and preimplantation genetic diagnosis (PGD) of embryos may drastically reduce the incidence of miscarriage, although its use is still in question in some circles and it is still very cost prohibitive, adding approximately $5000 to an IVF cycle.

Several studies have examined the link between sperm DNA damage levels and conception and miscarriage rates, so a systematic review and meta-analysis of studies which examined the effect of sperm DNA damage on miscarriage rates was performed. Sixteen cohort studies (2969 couples), 14 of which were prospective, showed a significant increase in miscarriage in patients with high DNA damage compared with those with low DNA damage. The researchers went on to express that the implications of these findings indicates that tests detecting DNA damage could be considered in those suffering from recurrent pregnancy loss. Further research is necessary to study the effects of damaged sperm DNA on fertility, and how the intake of dietary antioxidants improves sperm DNA and miscarriage rates (*Robinson, L. 2012*).

A study about the frequency of ejaculation and how it affects sperm's DNA concluded that shorter periods of abstinence between ejaculations displayed improvements in sperm DNA fragmentation. It should be noted that they

256

were comparing a group ejaculating every 24 hours with a group ejaculating every three hours, with three hours being the winner. The results of this study challenges the role of abstinence in current male infertility treatments and suggests that sperm DNA fragmentation can be efficiently reduced by a biological practice consisting of short-term recurrent ejaculation (*Gosálvez, 2011*).

If there is a link between poor sperm and miscarriage, then men should do everything they can to improve sperm parameters before trying to conceive, especially before jumping into IVF.

Chinese medicine has treated male infertility for a millennia. Most often I see very good results when the commitment is made.

Does poor sperm quality = poor embryo quality? Could poor sperm be getting women pregnant, but producing embryos of poor quality that do not live past the early weeks of pregnancy? It is an increasingly popular suggestion among healthcare professionals that men do everything they can to improve their overall health and sperm parameters before jumping into IVF or ICSI.

Supporting Your Partner

"If you love someone tell them...because hearts are often broken by words left unspoken."
~Pamela Daranjo

At any given time, I have at least two to three women who, as far as western medical testing is concerned, have absolutely nothing impairing their fertility. Time and again, I see women doing everything they can to better understand their circumstances and optimize their health, while the husband does nothing to improve his health and sperm or support his wife's efforts. This isn't right. It's a lot for a woman to take and hardly fair to her.

Supporting your partner during this time and taking responsibility for your role in creating a life is imperative not only to a healthy and happy relationship but I believe, to the success of conception. You want your partner and your future child to know that you were as much on-board with this pregnancy as was the person carrying the baby. A lack of participation may be causing stress to your partner during an already stressful time.

Make the lifestyle adaptations as recommended, go to as many doctor's appointments as possible, communicate about what you're feeling and listen to your partner. This is a chance to get closer if you allow it and excellent practice for the team building that makes for great parenting.

Through my own personal development and growth, I was able to recognize arrogance and fear in myself and am compassionate when I see it in other men. A great book that helped me a lot was 'The Way of the Superior Man' by David Deida. It will help you deeply understand how to really understand and succeed with women. He also wrote 'It's a Guy Thing - An Owner's Manual for Women.'

"Love is a Verb." ~Martin Luther King Jr.

Story
Jason R.

My wife Kristy and I have been married for almost a decade and started our journey towards having a child almost 6 years ago. At first we were able to get pregnant but each of four times ended in miscarriage; a devastating experience. Once we had seen a gauntlet of doctors, it was apparent that we would need some help in this process, which led us to fertility clinics.

The first clinic we went to was in late 2012. The process was overwhelming for both of us as we had never been through anything like it. Kristy was quite a trooper and like most males, I tried to always put on a brave front, often choosing to mourn privately so as to not add to Kristy's stress. It's funny how often we heard how lucky Kristy was to have my support. It seemed odd to me because I wouldn't have had it any other way. This was our future, our child, so it would always be our journey together as far as I was concerned. I don't think I did anything special; it's what every guy should be doing if he loves his wife and wants a child as badly as we did. Maybe some men don't think it's manly, but what could be more manly than supporting your wife?

During this time I started acupuncture. It was new to me but ultimately a rewarding experience that helped me become more of a relaxed person.

That first IVF was unsuccessful which really got us down for a couple of weeks. When we decided to try again, we went to a new clinic. Once again, we did it all together, from early morning ultrasounds, medication pickups, doctors' visits and acupuncture appointments. Kristy kept a brave face and handled it as well as one could expect. I, on the other hand, was starting to have irrational thoughts like we were being ripped off and that these doctors didn't know what they were doing. It was not good for my psyche but I guess it was a defense system trying to lay blame for the fact that natural parenthood may not be within our reach.

No matter how many times one goes through this process, it doesn't get easier. Our second IVF was also unsuccessful and having to relive the feeling of failure was not fun at all.

We decided to try a clinic in Seattle that came with a stellar reputation. This was also our only option to use an egg donor, since U.S. laws are a little less strict about it.

It was mid 2013 by then. I tried to stay strong for my wife. I often told her that if it was possible for me to do all the shots or take the pills that I would in a heartbeat. It was tough seeing her body put through so much and I wished I could do more.

Once again we were unsuccessful, but it was no easier. I'd almost come to expect failure, possibly to numb myself or try to prepare for the worst but it was still a major blow.

It was during this cycle that I stopped acupuncture and Kristy started seeing Dr. Pentland at Yinstill Reproductive Wellness. I guess one reason I quit going was that once again I felt that it was just a cash grab which while irrational is what my dark thoughts had me believing.

We decided that our next cycle would be our last as it had taken a toll on Kristy's body and been such a strain on our psyches. It was the realization that this was our last chance that really hit me hard. I couldn't mourn in private any longer. I found myself crying almost daily. It was as if all the disappointment of the last few years came flooding to the surface all at once. I finally let Kristy see how hard it was for me. I realized how badly I wanted to be a father.

We switched from Kristy's eggs to a donor's. This was not easy for her and it broke my heart to see her struggling with that decision, but as I always told her, "It's your body and only you truly know how you feel. Just know that I support any decision you feel most comfortable with". It was during this cycle that I myself started seeing Dr.

Pentland. Kristy had seen him during the last cycle and she thought it would be good for me to go back to help with my emotional struggles and it did. I definitely felt calmed and it was nice to have someone to talk to that understood.

The hardest part to swallow was the fact I'm insecure in many aspects of life, but I know with all my heart that I would make an excellent father. It's a type of confidence I've never had before. Having not had a father around growing up has only instilled a deep appreciation of what I would do for a child of mine and how much I would give. I really hope I get that chance.

Even at our lowest points, one thing I am grateful for is how close this has brought my wife and I. Many marriages are destroyed both emotionally and financially but this actually brought us together. Although we wanted children very badly, our focus was still always on each other and being a happy couple. We are truly blessed in so many ways and we keep reminding ourselves of that.

Update 1:

Our fourth round of In vitro was a success. It seems as if our 'small chance' was bigger than we thought. We are due in October 2014. There are no words to express how excited we are!

Update 2: October 2014 email from Kristy

Kaden is truly the one that was meant to be our child. I am loving every second of being a Mom, although he makes it easy to love him. When I heard his first cry in the delivery room it was worth every tear and heartache to get to that moment in our journey. We are so blessed to have him in our lives; he is just a wonderful little boy. He's not fussy, he just loves to be around us, our family and close friends. I just stare at him in amazement and feel so overwhelmed that our dream of being parents has come true. Thank you for your support thru our journey!

I feel confident that we are going to look back at this time in history and wonder why the male role in fertility was so under-emphasized when it is clearly such a large part of the baby-making equation. It's quite possible that one of the best ways to increase the chances of overcoming infertility, becoming pregnant, and having a healthy happy baby is to cultivate healthy men and healthy sperm.

Chapter Task:

List three simple ways you and/or your husband can help improve sperm quality right now:

1. _____

2. _____

3. _____

Write down any questions you still have about male reproductive health:

_____

_____

_____

_____

Now go and find answers to these questions!

<u>Conclusion</u>

I t is my sincere hope that this book has given you the necessary ingredients to create the recipe for a more fertile you.

Taking care of your health and well-being is the first priority once you have chosen to start a family. I hope I have provided a fuller understanding of Chinese Medicine as it relates to your reproductive health, and how it can help fulfill your dream of creating a happy, healthy family.

If you have not already done so, it is now time to go back to the end of each step and organize the chapter tasks into an action plan. Committing to this plan will help prepare your body mind and spirit for conception and a healthy pregnancy.

Once the plan is in place, work diligently to cultivate faith in the knowledge that you are taking the necessary steps toward 'being fertile' and that your body can do this, thereby surrendering and releasing yourself to enjoy life in the meantime.

The final and possibly most important ingredient left is to dig deep and find the strength required to persevere.

Think of this book as a tool for knowledge, support and cheerleading that you can refer to wherever you are on your path and share it with others that might need it.

My goal, and that of my truly amazing team at Yinstill, is to help as many people as we can to fulfill the dream of having a family. I speak from experience when I say nothing is more important. As my wife and I watch our boys grow, we are filled with gratitude and a love like no other. We want that for you too, so don't give up!

I wish you all the best creating your family.

Acknowledgments

I am blessed with so many wonderful people in my life that played a role in the manifestation of this book, but without a doubt **my beautiful wife Chantal** deserves my deepest gratitude and love. You have always been such an extraordinary support, far beyond expectation. You always believed in me and told me that I am a winner. You always inspire me to be my best, and just a little more, *'This little light of mine, I'm gonna let it shine!"* (Simon-Gervais). Thank you, my love. I am the luckiest man in the world.

AND in a close second are my two little dudes. I never knew that my heart could love SO much. Living each day knowing I am the primary example of a man in their life, understanding how that will shape and influence them, is all the motivation I need to be the best I can be. I am honored that you both chose me to be your dad. Words cannot express how much I love you, and how much I cherish every moment I get to spend with you. You taught me why the work I do is so important. I want everyone to experience what you have given me. Thank you, Salix and Ari.

My clients/patients, past and present. You have taught me so much, shared your souls with me. I am honoured that you chose me to be a part of your journey toward creating a family. I hope to never lose touch, as so many of you hold a very special place in my heart; you know who you are. I wish you and your family happiness and good health.

Thomas Kevin Dolan. You saved me, and guided me toward my potential. I would not have the life I do today if it wasn't for your wisdom, generosity and friendship. I do believe that you are an angel. Profound gratitude to the universe for manifesting Thomas in my life.

Rachael Biggs, thank you for all your help making this project happen. I am grateful for your contributions, skill in clarifying and editing my thoughts and messages, interviewing the wonderful women who offered their amazing stories, putting up with me and helping gift wrap this manuscript.

Dr. Harris Fisher & Dr. Erin Flynn. Your contributions and expertise are extremely appreciated. I am proud to work side-by-side. You all hold special places in the hearts of me and my family.

Blake Dobie, Natalie Villanueva, Claire Gondola, Rina Sidhu, Junko Lodge and Dr. Becky Stephens. Thank you all for all that you have done to help with this project.

Dr. Jeff Roberts, Dr. Jon Havelock and Dr. Sonya Kashyap. Thank you for taking the time to invite the integration of Chinese medicine into your practices, be open to how we can best serve our mutual patients, and develop friendships that have grown beyond mere professional connections.

To the many mentors and colleagues I have had the pleasure to spend time and study with over the years, thank you so very much. You have helped push me, support me and given me many tools to nurture my personal growth and to contribute to making the world a better place, something that I value very much in this lifetime. Honorable mention to Dr. Brown, my old friend. I want you to know that I miss you.

And last but not least, my mom, dad and brother, Ian (illustrator). You brought me into this world, gave me a safe loving place to grow up, and put up with me! I grow closer to you every day. I love you all so much, and miss you dearly. Sorry I have spent so much time so far away from you. To me, nothing is more important than family, so know that you are with me in my heart every day.

Sincerest gratitude, Spence

References

Avendaño, C., Franchi, A., Duran, H., & Oehninger, S. (2010). DNA fragmentation of normal spermatozoa negatively impacts embryo quality and intracytoplasmic sperm injection outcome. *Fertility and Sterility, 94*(2), 549-557.

Balercia, G., Buldreghini, E., Vignini, A., Tiano, L., Paggi, F., Amoroso, S., Littarru, G. (2009). Coenzyme Q10 treatment in infertile men with idiopathic asthenozoospermia: A placebo-controlled, double-blind randomized trial. *Fertility and Sterility, 91*(5), 1785-1792.

Belloc, S. (2014). Which Isolated Sperm Abnormality Is Most Related to Sperm DNA Damage in Men Presenting for Infertility Evaluation. *Journal of Assisted Reproduction and Genetics, 31*(5), 527-532.

Benrick, A. (2014). *Enhanced Insulin Sensitivity and Acute Regulation of Metabolic Genes and Signaling Pathways after a Single Electrical or Manual Acupuncture Session in Female Insulin-resistant Rats.* Acta Diabetologia.

Bhongade, M., Prasad, S., Jiloha, R., Ray, P., Mohapatra, S., & Koner, B. (n.d.). Effect of psychological stress on fertility hormones and seminal quality in male partners of infertile couples. *Andrologia,* doi: 10.1111/and.12268.

Boxmeer, J., Smit, M., Weber, R., Lindemans, J., Romijn, J., Eijkemans, M., Steegers-Theunissen, R. (2007). Seminal Plasma Cobalamin Significantly Correlates With Sperm Concentration in Men Undergoing IVF or ICSI Procedures. *Journal of Andrology,* 521-527.

Brown, E. (2013). *Unacceptable levels:* Pollution just got personal. Macroscopic Media.

Buck Louis, G. M., et al. (2013). Persistent Environmental Pollutants and Couple Fecundity: The LIFE Study. Environ Health Perspect. Retrieved from http://dx.doi.org/10.1289/ehp.1205301

Cakmak, Y., Akpinar, I., Ekinci, G., & Bekiroglu, N. (2008). Point- and frequency-specific response of the testicular artery to abdominal electroacupuncture in humans. *Fertility and Sterility, 90*(5), 1732-1738.

Chang-jie, S. (2007). An Integrated Chinese-Western Medical Treatment of 100 Cases of Male Oligospermia Sterility. *Heilongjiang Chinese Medicine & Pharmacology*, (3), 36-37.

Cheng, C. (2007). Observations on the Therapeutic Effects of Treating 132 Cases of Male Immune Infertility with Ju He Wan (Citrus Seed Pills). *Xin Zhong Yi (New Chinese Medicine)*, (7), 39-40.

Cheong, Y. et al. Acupuncture and Assisted Conception. *Cochrane Database of Systematic Reviews, 2008* (4).

Clarke, R. N. (1999). Relationship between Psychological Stress and Semen Quality among In-vitro Fertilization Patients. *Human Reproduction*, 14.3, 753-58.

Craig, L., Criniti, A., Hansen, K., Marshall, L., & Soules, M. (2007). Acupuncture lowers pregnancy rates when performed before and after embryo transfer. *Fertility and Sterility*, S40.

Dennis, N.A. et al. (2012). The level of serum anti-Müllerian hormone correlates with Vitamin D status in men and women but not in boys. *Journal of Clinical*

Endocrinology and Metabolism, (7), 2450-2455.

Dieterle, S. et al. (2009). A prospective randomized placebo-controlled study of the effect of acupuncture in infertile patients with severe oligoasthenozoospermia. *Fertility and Sterility*, 92(4), 1340–1343.

Donnelly, E., Lewis, S., Mcnally, J., & Thompson, W. (1998). In vitro fertilization and pregnancy rates: The influence of sperm motility and morphology on IVF outcome. *Fertility and Sterility*, 70(2), 305-314.

Estienne, M., Harper, A., & Crawford, R. (2008). Dietary supplementation with a source of omega-3 fatty acids increases sperm number and the duration of ejaculation in boars. *Theriogenology*, 70(1), 70-76.

Fiorani, M. & Magarelli, P. (n.d.). How Does Acupuncture Work? Scientific Western Explanation. Retrieved from: http://www.plantationacupuncture.org/#!acupuncture/c11c i

Fratterelli, J., Leondires, M., Fong, K., Theall, A., Locatelli, S., & Scott, R. (2008). Laser acupuncture before and after embryo transfer improves ART delivery rates: Results of a prospective randomized double-blinded placebo controlled five-armed trial involving 1000 patients. *Fertility and Sterility*, 90(Supp. 1), S105-S105.

Gennaro, L., Balistreri, S., Lenzi, A., Lombardo, F., Ferrara, M., & Gandini, L. (2003). Psychosocial factors discriminate oligozoospermic from normozoospermic men. *Fertility and Sterility*, (Supp. 3), 1571-1576.

Gerhard, I. (1992). Clinical data which influence semen parameters in infertile men. *Oxford Journals Human Reproduction*, 7(6).

Ghanbarzadeh, S. et al. (2013). Effects of L-Carnitine and Coenzyme Q10 on Impaired Spermatogenesis. Drug Research. Retrieved from http://www.ncbi.nlm.nih.gov/pubmed/24285403

Gleicher, N., & Barad, D. (2011). Dehydroepiandrosterone (DHEA) supplementation in diminished ovarian reserve (DOR). *Reproductive Biology and Endocrinology,* (9), 67.

Gollenberg, A., Liu, F., Brazil, C., Drobnis, E., Guzick, D., Overstreet, J., Swan, S. (2010). Semen quality in fertile men in relation to psychosocial stress. *Fertility and Sterility, 93*(4), 1104-1111.

Gosálvez, J., González-Martínez, M., López-Fernández, C., Fernández, J., & Sánchez-Martín, P. (2011). Shorter abstinence decreases sperm deoxyribonucleic acid fragmentation in ejaculate. *Fertility and Sterility, 96*(5), 1083-1086.

Hinks, J. (2010). An assessment of the demand and importance of acupuncture to patients of a fertility clinic during investigations and treatment. *Human Fertility, 13*(S1), 3-21.

Ishikawa, H. et al. (1996). Effects of Gui Zhi Fu Ling Wan on male infertility with varicocele. *American Journal of Chinese Medicine, 24*(3-4), 327-331.

Jeng, H. et al. (1997). A substance isolated from Cornus officinalis enhances the motility of human sperm. Department of Anatomy, Taipei Medical College, Taiwan. *American Journal of Chinese Medicine, 25*(3-4), 301-306.

Jensen, T. K. (2012). Association of Sleep Disturbances With Reduced Semen Quality: A Cross-sectional Study Among 953 Healthy Young Danish Men. *Oxford Journals*

American Journal of Epidemiology, 177(10), 1027-1037.

Kharrazian, D. (2010). Why Do I Still Have Thyroid Symptoms? When My Lab Tests Are Normal. Carlsbad CA: Elephant Press LP.

Khorram N. et al. (2012). Adjuvant acupuncture reduces first trimester pregnancy loss after IVF. Open Journal of Obstetrics and Gynecology. Retrieved from http://www.scirp.org/journal/ojog.

Kimmins, S. et al. (2013). Low paternal dietary folate alters the mouse sperm epigenome and is associated with negative pregnancy outcomes. Nature Communications.

Kinuta, K. (2000). Vitamin D Is an Important Factor in Estrogen Biosynthesis of Both Female and Male Gonads. *Endocrinology*, 1317-1324.

Kissell, K.A. et al. (2014). Biological variability in serum anti-Müllerian hormone throughout the menstrual cycle in ovulatory and sporadic anovulatory cycles in eumenorrheic women. *Oxford Journals Human Reproduction*.

Lafuente, R., González-Comadrán, M., Solà, I., López, G., Brassesco, M., Carreras, R., & Checa, M. (2013). Coenzyme Q10 and male infertility: A meta-analysis. *Journal of Assisted Reproduction and Genetics, 30*(9), 1147-1156.

Lai, A.N. et al. (1997). An experimental study on inhibitory effect of Chinese medicine tai-bao on antisperm antibody. *Chinese Journal of Integrated Traditional and Western Medicine. Zhongguo Zhong xi yi jie he xue hui, Zhongguo Zhong yi yan jiu yuan zhu ban, 17*(6), 360-362.

Lu, T.K. et al. (2006). Clinical study on the treatment of

male immune infertility. Hu zhang dan shen yin. Zhonghua Nan Ke Xue. *National Journal of Andrology,* *12*(8):750-755.

Lynch, C.D. et al. (2014). Preconception stress increases the risk of infertility: results from a couple-based prospective cohort study—the LIFE study. *Human Reproduction Oxford Journals.* (29)5.

Magarelli, P., Cridennda, D., & Cohen, M. (2009). Changes in serum cortisol and prolactin associated with acupuncture during controlled ovarian hyperstimulation in women undergoing in vitro fertilization–embryo transfer treatment. *Fertility and Sterility, 92*(6), 1870-1879.

Manheimer, E., Zhang, G., Udoff, L., Haramati, A., Langenberg, P., Berman, B., & Bouter, L. (2012). Effects of acupuncture on rates of pregnancy and live birth among women undergoing in vitro fertilisation: Systematic review and meta-analysis. *BMJ,* 545-549.

Manheimer, E., Windt, D., Cheng, K., Stafford, K., Liu, J., Tierney, J., Bouter, L. (2013). The effects of acupuncture on rates of clinical pregnancy among women undergoing in vitro fertilization: A systematic review and meta-analysis. *Human Reproduction Update,* 696-713.

Mendiola, J., Torres-Cantero, A., Moreno-Grau, J., Ten, J., Roca, M., Moreno-Grau, S., & Bernabeu, R. (2009). Food intake and its relationship with semen quality: A case-control study. *Fertility and Sterility, 91*(3), 812-818.

Mitchell, M., Bakos, H., & Lane, M. (2011). Paternal diet-induced obesity impairs embryo development and implantation in the mouse. *Fertility and Sterility, 95*(4), 1349-1353.

Muthusami, K., & Chinnaswamy, P. (2005). Effect Of

Chronic Alcoholism On Male Fertility Hormones And Semen Quality. *Fertility and Sterility, 84*(4), 919-924.

Pei, J., Strehler, E., Noss, U., Abt, M., Piomboni, P., Baccetti, B., & Sterzik, K. (2005). Quantitative evaluation of spermatozoa ultrastructure after acupuncture treatment for idiopathic male infertility. *Fertility and Sterility, 84*(1), 141-147.

Porpora, M., Brunelli, R., Costa, G., Imperiale, L., Krasnowska, E., Lundeberg, T., Parasassi, T. (2013). A Promise in the Treatment of Endometriosis: An Observational Cohort Study on Ovarian Endometrioma Reduction by N-Acetylcysteine. *Evidence-based Complementary and Alternative Medicine,* (Article ID 240702), 1-7.

Robinson, L., Gallos, I., Conner, S., Rajkhowa, M., Miller, D., Lewis, S., Coomarasamy, A. (2012). The effect of sperm DNA fragmentation on miscarriage rates: A systematic review and meta-analysis. *Human Reproduction, 27*(10), 2908-2917.

Safarinejad, M. (2011). Effect of omega-3 polyunsaturated fatty acid supplementation on semen profile and enzymatic anti-oxidant capacity of seminal plasma in infertile men with idiopathic oligoasthenoteratospermia: A double-blind, placebo-controlled, randomised study. *Andrologia, 43*(1), 38-47.

Safarinejad, R.M. et al. (2010). Relationship of omega-3 and omega-6 fatty acids with semen characteristics, and anti-oxidant status of seminal plasma: A comparison between fertile and infertile men. *Clinical Nutrition, 29*(1), 100-105.

Shayeb, A.G. et al. (2011). An exploration of the association between male body mass index and semen quality. Reproductive BioMedicine Online, *23*(6), 717–723.

Shirley, R.L. et al. (1963). Effect of Dietary Protein on Fructose, Citric Acid and 5-Nucleotidase Activity in the Semen of Bulls. *Journal of Animal Science, 22*, 14-18.

Siterman S. et al. (1997). Effect of acupuncture on sperm parameters of males suffering from subfertility related to low sperm quality. Archives of Andrology, *39*(2), 155-1561.

Siterman S. et al. (2009). Acupuncture Helps Lower Scrotum Temperature, Increase Sperm Count. *Asian Journal of Andrology, 11*(2), 200-208.

Siterman, S., Eltes, F., Wolfson, V., Lederman, H., & Bartoov, B. (2000). Does acupuncture treatment affect sperm density in males with very low sperm count? A pilot study. *Andrologia 32*(1), 31-39.

Stener-Victorin, E., Kobayashi, R., & Kurosawa, M. (2003). Ovarian blood flow responses to electro-acupuncture stimulation at different frequencies and intensities in anaesthetized rats. *Autonomic Neuroscience, 108*(1-2), 50-56.

Stener-Victorin, E., Waldenstrom, U., Andersson, S., & Wikland, M. (1996). Reduction of blood flow impedance in the uterine arteries of infertile women with electro-acupuncture. *Human Reproduction, 11*, 1314-1317.

Sun Z. et al. (2006). TCM treatment of male immune infertility--a report of 100 cases. *Journal of Traditional Chinese Medicine, 26*(1), 36-38.

Turner, K. et al. (2013). Stress and Anxiety Scores in First and Repeat IVF Cycles. PLOS ONE, *8*(5).

Turunen, M., Olsson, J., & Dallner, G. (2004). Metabolism and function of coenzyme Q. *Biochimica Et Biophysica Acta (BBA) - Biomembranes,* (1660), 171-199.

Vellani, E., Colasante, A., Mamazza, L., Minasi, M., Greco, E., & Bevilacqua, A. (2013). Association of state and trait anxiety to semen quality of in vitro fertilization patients: A controlled study. *Fertility and Sterility, 99*(6), 1565-1572.e2.

Vujkovic, M. et al. (2009). Associations between dietary patterns and semen quality in men undergoing IVF/ICSI treatment. Human Reproduction, Oxford Journals.

Wang, S. J. et al. (2014). Acupuncture relieves the excessive excitation of hypothalamic-pituitary-adrenal cortex axis function and correlates with the regulatory mechanism of GR, CRH and ACTHR. *Evidence-Based Complementary and Alternative Medicine.* Retrieved from http://www.pubfacts.com/detail/24761151/Acupuncture-Relieves-the-Excessive-Excitation-of-Hypothalamic-Pituitary-Adrenal-Cortex-Axis-Function.

Wong, W., Merkus, H., Thomas, C., Menkveld, R., Zielhuis, G., & Steegers-Theunissen, R. (2002). Effects of folic acid and zinc sulfate on male factor subfertility: A double-blind, randomized, placebo-controlled trial. *Fertility and Sterility, 77*(3), 491-498.

Wynter, K., Mcmahon, C., Hammarberg, K., Mcbain, J., Boivin, J., Gibson, F., & Fisher, J. (2013). Spontaneous conceptions within two years of having a first infant with assisted conception. *Australian and New Zealand Journal of Obstetrics and Gynaecology, 53*(5), 471–476.

Yamanaka, M. et al. (1998). Direct effects of Chinese herbal medicine "hachuekkito" on sperm movement. A Department of Urology, Osaka University Medical School

- Nippon Hinyokika Gakkai Zasshi, *89*(7), 641-646.

Yue, G.P. et al. (1996). Male infertility treated by bu shen sheng jing pill in clinical observation and evaluation on its curative effect. *Chinese Journal of Integrated Traditional and Western Medicine. Zhongguo Zhong xi yi jie he xue hui, Zhongguo Zhong yi yan jiu yuan zhu ban, 16*(8), 463-466.

Zareba, P., Colaci, D., Afeiche, M., Gaskins, A., Jørgensen, N., Mendiola, J., Chavarro, J. (2013). Semen quality in relation to antioxidant intake in a healthy male population. *Fertility and Sterility, 100*(6), 1572-1579.

Zhang M. et al. (2002). Influence of acupuncture on idiopathic male infertility in assisted reproductive technology. *Journal of Huazhong University Science Technology Med Sci, 22*(3), 228-230.

Zhang, J. et al. (2008). The Treatment of 156 Cases of Oligospermia with Sheng Jing Qiang You Tang (Engender Essence & Strengthen Fertility Decoction). *Shi Yong Zhong Yi Nei Ke Za Zhi (Journal of Practical Chinese Medical Internal Medicine)*, (1), 50.

Zheng, C., Huang, G., Zhang, M., & Wang, W. (2012). Effects of acupuncture on pregnancy rates in women undergoing in vitro fertilization: A systematic review and meta-analysis. *Fertility and Sterility, 97*(3), 599-611.

Zhou, K. et al. (2013). Acupuncture changes reproductive hormone levels in patients with ovarian deficiency - prospective observational study. *Evidence-Based Complementary Alternative Medicine.* Retrieved from http://www.pubfacts.com/detail/23533511/Electroacupuncture-modulates-reproductive-hormone-levels-in-patients-with-primary-ovarian-insufficie

Glossary

The following definitions/explanations are excerpted from Wikipedia.

Androgens - Broad term for any natural or synthetic compound, usually a steroid hormone, that stimulates or controls the development and maintenance of male characteristics in vertebrates by binding to androgen receptors. Androgens are the precursor of all estrogens. The primary and most well-known androgen is testosterone.

Andrology - The medical specialty that deals with male health, particularly relating to the problems of the male reproductive system and urological problems that are unique to men. It is also known as "The science of Men." It is the counterpart to gynecology.

Antimullerian hormone (AMH) - AMH is expressed by granulosa cells of the ovary during the reproductive years, and limits the formation of primary follicles by inhibiting excessive follicular recruitment by FSH. Some authorities suggest it is a measure of certain aspects of ovarian function, useful in assessing conditions such as polycystic ovary syndrome and premature ovarian failure. It is useful to predict a poor ovarian response in in vitro fertilization (IVF), but it does not appear to add any predictive information about success rates of an already established pregnancy after IVF.

Antioxidant - A molecule (commonly found in colourful plants and dietary supplements) that inhibits the oxidation of other molecules (within cells and tissues of the body). Oxidation produces free radicals. These radicals can start chain reactions. When the chain reaction occurs in a cell, it can cause damage or death to the cell. Antioxidants terminate these chain reactions by removing free radicals and inhibiting other oxidation reactions.

Antral Follicle Count (AFC) - The number of antral follicles (ovarian follicle during a certain latter stage of folliculogenesis) in both ovaries, determined by transvaginal ultrasonography.

Assisted reproductive technologies (ART) - Methods used to achieve pregnancy by artificial or partially artificial means. It is reproductive technology used primarily for infertility treatments, and is also known as fertility treatment.

ATP (Adenosine triphosphate) - Coenzyme used as an energy carrier in the cells of all known organisms; the process in which energy is moved throughout the cell.

Basal body temperature (BBT) - The lowest body temperature attained, generally measured immediately after awakening and before any physical activity has been undertaken. Monitoring of BBTs is one way of estimating the day of ovulation. The tendency of a woman to have lower temperatures before ovulation and higher temperatures afterwards, is known as a biphasic pattern. Charting of this pattern may be used as a component of fertility awareness.

Biomarker - A measurable indicator of the severity or presence of some disease state. More generally a biomarker is anything that can be used as an indicator of a particular disease state or some other physiological state of an organism.

Blastocyst - A structure formed in the early development of mammals which subsequently forms the embryo. The outer layer of the blastocyst consists of cells collectively called the trophoblast. The trophoblast gives rise to the placenta. In humans, blastocyst formation begins about 5 days after fertilization. The blastocyst has a diameter of about 0.1-0.2 mm and comprises 200-300 cells following rapid cleavage (cell division). After about 1 day, the blastocyst implants itself into the endometrium of the uterine wall.

Body Mass Index (BMI) - A measure of relative weight based on an individual's mass and height.

Candida - Candidiasis, thrush, or yeast infection is a fungal infection (mycosis) which encompasses infections that range from superficial (such as oral thrush and vaginitis) to systemic and more severe conditions. Superficial infections of the skin and mucosal membranes cause local inflammation and discomfort.

Casein - Proteins which are commonly found in mammalian milk, making up 80% of the proteins in cow milk and between 20% and 45% of the proteins in human milk.

Cortisol - A steroid hormone, more specifically a glucocorticoid, which is produced by the adrenal glands. It is released in response to stress and a low level of blood glucose. Its functions are to increase blood sugar through gluconeogenesis, to suppress the immune system, and to aid the metabolism of fat, protein and carbohydrate. It also decreases bone formation.

Cyst - A cluster of cells that have grouped together to form a sac (not unlike the manner in which water molecules group together, forming a bubble); however, the distinguishing aspect of a cyst is the cells forming the "shell" of such a sac are distinctly abnormal (in both appearance and behaviour) when compared to all surrounding cells for that given location.

D&C (dilation or dilatation and curettage) - Dilation (widening/opening) of the cervix and surgical removal of part of the lining of the uterus and/or contents of the uterus by scraping and scooping (curettage). It is a therapeutic gynecological procedure as well as the most often used method of first trimester pregnancy loss and abortion.

DHA (Docosahexaenoic acid) - An Omega-3 fatty acid (most often obtained from fish) that is a primary structural component of the human brain, cerebral cortex, skin, sperm, testicles and retina. It can be synthesized from alpha-linolenic acid or obtained directly from maternal milk or fish oil. Important for the developing fetus and healthy breast milk.

DHEA (dehydoepiandosterone) - Is the most abundant circulating steroid hormone in humans, in whom it is produced in the adrenal glands, the gonads and the brain, where it functions predominantly as a metabolic intermediate in the biosynthesis of the androgen and estrogen sex steroids.

Diminished ovarian reserve (DOR) - Also known as poor ovarian reserve, impaired ovarian reserve, premature ovarian aging or declining ovarian reserve, is a condition of low fertility characterized by 1): low numbers of remaining oocytes in the ovaries or 2): possibly impaired preantral oocyte development or recruitment.

Dioxin - Dioxin and dioxin-like compounds (DLCs) are by-products of various industrial processes and are commonly regarded as highly toxic compounds that are environmental pollutants and persistent organic pollutants (POPs). They include: Polychlorinated dibenzo-p-dioxins (PCDDs), or simply dioxins. Polychlorinated dibenzofurans (PCDFs) and Polychlorinated biphenyls (PCBs) have "dioxin-like" properties.

Endocrinology - A branch of biology and medicine dealing with the endocrine system, its diseases and its specific secretions called hormones, as well as the integration of developmental events proliferation, growth, and differentiation (including histogenesis and organogenesis), and also the psychological or behavioral activities of metabolism, growth and development, tissue function, sleep, digestion, respiration, excretion, mood, stress, lactation, movement, reproduction and sensory perception as caused by hormones. Endocrinology is concerned with study of the biosynthesis, storage, chemistry, biochemical and physiological function of hormones and with the cells of the endocrine glands and tissues that secrete them. Various specializations exist, including behavioral endocrinology and comparative endocrinology. The endocrine system consists of several glands, all in different parts of the body, that secrete hormones directly into the blood rather than into a duct system. Hormones have many different functions and modes of action; one hormone may have several effects on different target organs, and, conversely, one target organ may be affected by more than one hormone.

Endometriosis - A hormonal and immune system disease in which cells similar to that which line the uterus (endometrium) grow outside the uterine cavity, most commonly on the membrane which lines the abdominal cavity, the peritoneum. The uterine cavity is lined with endometrial cells, which are under the influence of female hormones. Endometrial cells in areas outside the uterus are also influenced by hormonal changes and respond in a way that is similar to the cells found inside the uterus. Common symptoms of endometriosis are pain and infertility. The pain often is worse with the menstrual cycle and is the most common cause of secondary dysmenorrhea.

EPA (Eicosapentaenoic acid) - An Omega-3 polyunsaturated fatty acid most often obtained from fish. It acts as a precursor for prostaglandin-3 (which inhibits platelet aggregation) and has the ability to reduce inflammation.

Estrogen(s) - A group of compounds named for their importance in both menstrual and estrous reproductive cycles. They are the primary female sex hormones.

Femoral massage - Compression of the large femoral artery palpable in the groin between the lower abdomen and the upper thigh. It is intended to increase supply of blood flow to the uterus, fallopian tubes and ovaries.

Fibroid (uterine) - A leiomyoma (benign tumor from smooth muscle tissue) that originates from the smooth muscle layer (myometrium) of the uterus.

Flora (gut) - More appropriately, gut microbiota, consists of a complex of microorganism species that live in the digestive tracts of animals. Gut microorganisms benefit the host by gleaning the energy from the fermentation of undigested carbohydrates, the subsequent absorption of short-chain fatty acids (butyrates, propionates, acetates), and play a role in synthesizing Vitamin B and Vitamin K, and metabolising bile acids, sterols and xenobiotics.

Folliculogenesis - The maturation life cycle of an ovarian follicle (shell on ovary which contains an immature egg).

Follicle-stimulating hormone (FSH) - A hormone secreted by the anterior pituitary gland. FSH regulates the development, growth, pubertal maturation and reproductive processes of the body.

Gluten - A protein composite found in wheat and related grains, including barley and rye. Gluten gives elasticity to dough, helping it rise and keep its shape and often gives the final product a chewy texture. Gluten is used in cosmetics, hair products and other dermatological preparations.

Gonadotropins - Follicle-stimulating hormone (FSH), luteinizing hormone (LH), placental chorionic gonadotropins hCG and eCG and chorionic gonadotropin

(CG). These protein hormones are central to the complex endocrine system that regulates normal growth, sexual development and reproductive function. The hormones LH and FSH are secreted by the anterior pituitary gland, while hCG and eCG are secreted by the placenta.

Hashimoto's thyroiditis - An autoimmune disease in which the thyroid gland is attacked by a variety of cell- and antibody-mediated immune processes. It was the first disease to be recognized as an autoimmune disease.

Holistic - The idea that natural systems (physical, biological, chemical, social, economic, mental, linguistic, etc.) and their properties should be viewed as wholes, not as collections of parts. This often includes the view that systems function as wholes and that their functioning cannot be fully understood solely in terms of their component parts.

Homocysteine - A non-protein a-amino acid. A high level of homocysteine in the blood (hyperhomocysteinemia) makes a person more prone to endothelial cell injury, which leads to inflammation in the blood vessels, cardiovascular disease, miscarriage and polycystic ovary syndrome (PCOS). Homocysteine can be converted into methionine or converted into cysteine with the aid of B-vitamins.

Hyperthyroidism - Often called overactive thyroid, a condition in which the thyroid gland produces and secretes excessive amounts of the free (not protein bound circulating in the blood) thyroid hormones - triiodothyronine (T3) and/or thyroxine (T4). Graves' disease is the most common cause of hyperthyroidism. The opposite is hypothyroidism.

Hypothyroidism - Often called underactive thyroid or low thyroid, is a common endocrine disorder in which the thyroid gland does not produce enough thyroid hormone.

The diagnosis of hypothyroidism can be confirmed with blood tests measuring thyroid-stimulating hormone (TSH) and thyroxine levels. The opposite is Hyperthyroidism.

Hysterosalpingogram (HSG) - A radiologic imaging procedure to investigate the shape of the uterine cavity and the shape and patency of the fallopian tubes. It entails the injection of a radio-opaque material into the cervical canal and usually fluoroscopy with image intensification. A normal result shows the filling of the uterine cavity and the bilateral filling of the fallopian tube with the injection material.

In Vitro Fertilization (IVF) - A process by which an egg is fertilised by sperm outside the body: in vitro ("in glass"). The process involves monitoring and stimulating a woman's ovulatory process, removing ovum or ova (egg or eggs) from the woman's ovaries and letting sperm fertilise them in a fluid medium in a laboratory. The fertilised egg (zygote) is cultured for 2–6 days in a growth medium and is then implanted in the same or another woman's uterus, with the intention of establishing a successful pregnancy.

Inflammation - A protective attempt by the organism to remove the injurious stimuli and to initiate the healing process. Inflammation is not a synonym for infection, even though the two are often correlated (the former often being a result of the latter). The classical signs of acute inflammation are pain, heat, redness, swelling and loss of function.

Inositol - Helps balance blood sugar levels via insulin signal transduction. Inositol (Vitamin B8) is a carbohydrate, though not a classical sugar. It has a taste which has been assayed at half the sweetness of table sugar (sucrose).

Intracytoplasmic sperm injection (ICSI) - An in vitro

fertilization procedure in which a single sperm is injected directly into an egg.

IUD (Intrauterine device) - A small contraceptive device, often 'T'-shaped, often containing either copper or levonorgestrel, which is inserted into the uterus. They are one form of long-acting reversible contraceptions which are the most effective types of reversible birth control.

Karyotype - Describes the number of chromosomes, and what they look like under a light microscope. Attention is paid to their length, the position of the centromeres, banding pattern, any differences between the sex chromosomes and any other physical characteristics. The preparation and study of karyotypes is part of cytogenetics.

Laparoscopy - An operation performed in the abdomen or pelvis through small incisions (usually 0.5–1.5 cm) with the aid of a camera. It can either be used to inspect and diagnose a condition or to perform surgery.

Luteinizing hormone (LH) - A hormone produced by gonadotroph cells in the anterior pituitary gland. In females, an acute rise of LH ("LH surge") triggers ovulation and development of the corpus luteum. In males, it stimulates Leydig cell production of testosterone. It acts synergistically with FSH.

Menarche - The first menstrual cycle, or first menstrual bleeding, in female humans. From both social and medical perspectives, it is often considered the central event of female puberty, as it signals the possibility of fertility.

Mitochondria - A membrane bound organelle found in most eukaryotic cells (the cells that make up plants, animals, fungi and many other forms of life) sometimes described as "cellular power plants" because they generate most of the cell's supply of adenosine triphosphate (ATP), used as a source of chemical energy.

Myofascial release - A soft tissue therapy for the treatment of skeletal muscle immobility and pain. This alternative medicine therapy aims to relax contracted muscles, improve blood and lymphatic circulation and stimulate the stretch reflex in muscles.

Neuromuscular therapy (NMT) - An approach to soft tissue manual therapy in which quasi-static pressure is applied to soft tissue to stimulate skeletal striated muscle. Often these areas of muscle are myofascial trigger points. NMT practitioners claim to balance the central nervous system (brain, spinal column and nerves) with the structure and form of the musculoskeletal system. Through applied knowledge of trigger points, neuromuscular therapy addresses postural distortion (poor posture), biomechanical dysfunction, nerve compression syndrome and ischemia.

Nocturia - Is defined by the International Continence Society (ICS) as "the complaint that the individual has to wake at night one or more times for voiding."

PCB (Polychlorinated biphenyl) - A synthetic organic chemical compound of chlorine attached to biphenyl, which is a molecule composed of two benzene rings. Polychlorinated biphenyls were widely used as dielectric and coolant fluids, for example in electrical apparatus, cutting fluids for machining operations, carbon paper and in heat transfer fluids. Due to PCBs' environmental toxicity and classification as a persistent organic pollutant, PCB production was banned by the United States Congress in 1979 and by the Stockholm Convention on Persistent Organic Pollutants in 2001.

Polycystic Ovary Syndrome (PCOS) - Also called hyperandrogenic anovulation (HA), or Stein-Leventhal syndrome, is one of the most common endocrine disorders among women. PCOS has a diverse range of causes that are not entirely understood, but there is evidence that it is largely a genetic disease. Others say it is generally a metabolic dysfunction, since it is reversible. Even though the name suggests that the ovaries are the cornerstone of disease pathology, cysts are the 'result' , not the cause of the disease. Gynecologists often see it as a gynecological problem, with the ovary as the primary organ affected. However, recent insights shows a multisystem disorder, with the primary problems lying in hormonal regulation in hypothalamus, with involvement of many organs. Treatments like wedge resection or laparoscopic drilling of ovaries are still performed around the world, based on this false 'ovary-focused' belief. It is thought to be one of the leading causes of female subfertility and the most frequent endocrine problem in women of reproductive age. The most common immediate symptoms are anovulation, excess androgenic hormones and insulin resistance. Anovulation results in irregular menstruation, amenorrhea and ovulation-related infertility. Hormone imbalance generally causes acne and hirsutism. Insulin resistance is associated with obesity, Type 2 diabetes and high cholesterol levels. The symptoms and severity of the syndrome vary greatly among those affected.

Polyp - An endometrial polyp or uterine polyp is a mass in the inner lining of the uterus. They may have a large flat base (sessile) or be attached to the uterus by an elongated pedicle (pedunculated). Pedunculated polyps are more common than sessile. They range in size from a few millimeters to several centimeters.

Preimplantation genetic diagnosis (PGD) - Genetic profiling of embryos prior to implantation. PGD is considered in a similar fashion to prenatal diagnosis. When used to screen for a specific genetic disease, its main advantage is that it avoids selective pregnancy termination, as the method makes it highly likely that the baby will be free of the disease under consideration. PGD thus is an adjunct to assisted reproductive technology, and requires in vitro fertilization (IVF) to obtain oocytes or embryos for evaluation.

Probiotics - The World Health Organization's 2001 definition of probiotics is 'live micro-organisms which, when administered in adequate amounts, confer a health benefit on the host.'

Progesterone (P4) - An endogenous steroid hormone involved in the menstrual cycle, pregnancy and embryogenesis of humans and other species.

Qigong - Chi kung, or chi gung (literally: "Life Energy Cultivation") is a practice of aligning body, breath and mind for health, meditation and martial arts training. With roots in Chinese medicine, philosophy and martial arts, qigong is traditionally viewed as a practice to cultivate and balance qi (chi) or what has been translated as "life energy".

Reductionism - Modern bioscientific position that holds that a complex system is nothing but the sum of its parts, and that an account of it can be reduced to accounts of individual constituents.

RPL (recurrent pregnancy loss) - RPL, or recurrent miscarriage, is the occurrence of three or more consecutive pregnancies that end in miscarriage of the fetus before viability.

Spermatogenesis - The process in which sperm are produced.

Uterine lining - Uterine lining, or, endometrium, is the inner mucous membrane of the uterus.

Vaginal pH - A measure of the acidity or basicity of vaginal fluids. A pH less than 7 is said to be acidic and a pH greater than 7 are basic or alkaline. Pure water has a pH very close to 7.

Varicocele - An abnormal enlargement of veins in the

scrotum.

Visceral manipulation - A physical treatment primarily used by massage therapists for conditions of the abdominal organs; it most commonly includes kneading and manipulation of the abdomen.

Volatile organic compound (VOC) - Organic chemicals that have a high vapor pressure at ordinary room temperature. Their high vapor pressure results from a low boiling point, which causes large numbers of molecules to evaporate or sublimate from the liquid or solid form of the compound and enter the surrounding air. They include both human-made and naturally occurring chemical compounds. Most scents or odours are of VOCs. VOCs play an important role in communication between plants and messages from plants to animals. Some VOCs are dangerous to human health or cause harm to the environment. Anthropogenic VOCs are regulated by law, especially indoors, where concentrations are the highest. Harmful VOCs typically are not acutely toxic, but have compounding long-term health effects. Because the concentrations are usually low and the symptoms slow to develop, research into VOCs and their effects is difficult.

Vulvodynia - A chronic pain syndrome that affects the vulvar area and occurs without an identifiable cause. Symptoms typically include a feeling of burning or irritation. The exact cause is unknown but is believed to involve a number of factors, including genetics, immunology and possibly diet. Diagnosis is by ruling out other possible causes.

Y chromosome microdeletion (YCM) - A family of genetic disorders caused by missing gene(s) in the Y chromosome. Many men with YCM exhibit no symptoms and lead normal lives. However, YCM is also known to be present in a significant number of men with reduced fertility. Men with reduced sperm production (in up to

20% of men with reduced sperm count, some form of YCM has been detected) varies from oligozoospermia, significant lack of sperm, or azoospermia, complete lack of sperm.

Index

treatment of Qi of the
kidneys, 26
Winfrey, Oprah, 71, 200
Woodhouse, Natalie, 184-87
The World Health
    Organization (WHO), 122

X
Xenoestrogens, 118

Y
Yager, Holly, 174-76
Yang Deficiency (Cold), 24
    examples of, 24-25
    features of, 24
    food cures for, 134-35
    kidney yang, 250
Yearwood, Trisha, 97
Yin Deficiency, 21
    examples of, 22-24,
    features of, 21-22
    food cures for, 142-43
Yinstill [Reproductive
    Wellness], 2, 185
    Gratitude Forest, 4
Yintang acupressure, 178
Yoga, 30, 55-57, 60, 223, 249,
252

Z
Zinc, 237

41190842R00189

Made in the USA
Charleston, SC
25 April 2015